#1 INTERNATIO

CARDIAC FAILURE

Explained

Dr Warrick Bishop
with Penelope Edman

SCAN FOR BONUSES

CARDIAC FAILURE

Explained

UNDERSTANDING THE SYMPTOMS, SIGNS, MEDICAL TESTS, AND MANAGEMENT OF A FAILING HEART

This book is for you, if you

- suffer from cardiac failure or know someone who does
- want to know what's going on with your heart
- need to know that you are not alone
- come from a family with 'bad' hearts
- are a carer of someone with cardiac failure
- want to understand the condition
- believe that understanding assists with better management
- would enjoy an informative read about an increasingly common condition
- are a medical, nursing or other health professional student wanting a 'taster' on the complexities of cardiac failure
- are a doctor requiring a straight-forward refresher or a book you can recommend to your patients

This book is also for you if you have a heart.

PUBLISHER'S NOTE

The author and editors of this publication have made every effort to provide information that is accurate and complete as of the date of publication. Readers are advised not to rely on the information provided without consulting their own medical advisers. It is the responsibility of the reader's treating physician or specialist, who relies on experience and knowledge about the patient, to determine the condition of, and the best treatment for, the reader. The information contained in this publication is provided without warranty of any kind. The author and editors disclaim responsibility for any errors, mis-statements, typographical errors or omissions in this publication.

National Library of Australia Cataloguing-in-Publication entry

Author:	Dr Warrick Bishop
Website:	www.drwarrickbishop.com
Website:	www.healthyheartnetwork.com
With:	Penelope Edman, *PAGE 56*
Title:	Cardiac Failure Explained
ISBN:	978-0-6452681-0-2 Amazon Paperback
ISBN:	978-0-6452681-1-9 Paperback
ISBN:	978-0-6452681-2-6 Hardcover
ASIN:	B096VBSKV3 Amazon eBook
ISBN:	978-0-6452681-3-3 (eBook)
Subject:	Cardiac health care
Publisher:	Dr Warrick Bishop
Designer:	Cathy McAuliffe, *Cathy McAuliffe Design*
Illustrator:	Cathy McAuliffe, *Cathy McAuliffe Design*

Interior V9

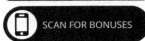

SCAN FOR BONUSES

For Book Bonuses visit https://drwarrickbishop.com/page/cardiacbookbonus

Dedicated to
DAVE.
Friends always.

CONTENTS

foreword 8

references 10

introduction   a defining conversation 13

THE HEART, SOME BASIC UNDERSTANDINGS

chapter 1   a high-functioning engine 21

              a closer look - the components of the heart 25

chapter 2   body pumps, pipes and regulators 35

              a closer look - understanding cardiac output................. 40

chapter 3   close neighbors..49

              patient's perspective: Terry's journey.............................. 55

chapter 4   challenging the body's fluid balance................................ 57

THE HEART, WHEN IT FAILS

              patient's perspective: Emma's journey 73

              a closer look - cardiac failure at a glance 77

chapter 5   short of breath? puffy ankles? 79

chapter 6   causes of cardiac failure 85

              case study —Barney 90

              case study — Freddy.. 97

chapter 7   diagnosis and investigation 101

chapter 8   more specific tests 109

THE HEART, CARDIAC FAILURE TREATMENT

              case study — Kathleen.......................................119

              patient's perspective: Kathleen's journey 123

chapter 9   treatment — an overview 127

chapter 10   drugs – diuretics 133

chapter 11   drugs – ACE inhibitors 141

chapter 12   drugs – AT2 receptor blockers 147

              a closer look - bilateral renal artery stenosis 149

              a closer look - NSAIDs.. 151

chapter 13   drugs – beta-blockers 155

chapter 14   drugs – next line...159

               case study – Martin... 162

chapter 15   implanted devices and surgical procedures................... 169

               case study – Barry...174

               patient's perspective: Gordon's journey..................... 184

chapter 16   common partners...191

               case study – Charlie 193

               *a closer look - the psychological aspects associated
               with cardiac failure* 199

chapter 17   acute cardiac failure.....................................205

               a closer look - 'Takotsubo' 210

THE HEART, LIVING WITH CARDIAC FAILURE

chapter 18   management of cardiac failure – a holistic approach......217

               patient's perspective: Cam's journey 219

chapter 19   lifestyle.. 221

chapter 20   women 231

               case study – Jill... 235

chapter 21   doctor, can I?...239

epilogue   beyond the horizon 249

appendix 1   drugs of cardiac failure 254

               timelines 256

               action of agents 258

appendix 2   understanding the QRS complex 260

appendix 3   consensus statement: definition, classification (2021)...266

list of illustrations, tables and photographs 272

glossary.. 274

index 285

thanks 291

about the authors 293

FOREWORD

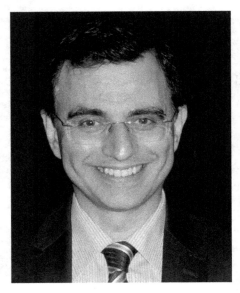

Heart failure is a very common syndrome affecting approximately 480,000 people in Australia and more than 25 million world-wide. It is the Cinderella of cardiovascular disease. It much less well known than heart attack or stroke, yet heart failure is a serious condition with a worse outcome than most cancers. Historically, more than half of the people diagnosed with heart failure would not survive five years. Thankfully, this situation is improving.

Heart failure is the end-product of a number of other conditions, such as heart attack, difficult to control blood pressure, hereditary factors, heart valve issues, toxins to the heart, or viral illnesses, among many others. Yet, regardless of the origin, it causes typical symptoms of fatigue, breathlessness, loss of appetite, swelling of the legs, bloating and the inability to do the things with which one could previously cope. In fact, heart failure causes a worse quality of life than chronic lung disease, chronic arthritis, angina, diabetes and high blood pressure. This often leads to hospitalizations, and in some cases, multiple hospitalizations, so-called 'frequent flyers'. Such hospitalizations cause heavy economic burden on the health system. Heart failure actually leads to the highest cardiac length of stay in hospital and is the most common cardiovascular cause of readmission to hospital. It costs the Australian health budget over two billion dollars per year.

So, heart failure is common, it kills you, it makes you feel bad and it costs lots of money! Fortunately, there are many things that can now improve outcomes for people who have heart failure, and these are outlined in this excellent book.

We are lucky that there has been a great deal of research into heart failure in the past 30 years. There are now many medicines which can improve survival, reduce hospitalization and improve symptoms for this serious condition and Warrick Bishop has explained these beautifully. We have also developed improved systems of care with help from heart failure nurses, physiotherapists, occupational therapists, pharmacists, social workers, psychologists, all with the patient as the central focus of care. These advancements have been summarized in the *Australian Guidelines for the Prevention, Detection and Management of Heart Failure*, of which I was fortunate to have been a co-author.

There is still a great deal to achieve in improving symptoms and survival outcomes in people who have heart failure. If we apply the principles described by Warrick, then it will be a great start. Most importantly, *Cardiac Failure Explained* informs patients. It also is an easy read for medical students and nurses who are learning about this condition, and it is a comprehensive refresher for general practitioners. Remember, knowledge is power and this is, therefore, a powerful book.

PROFESSOR ANDREW SINDONE

Director, Heart Failure Unit and Department of Cardiac Rehabilitation, Concord Hospital, Sydney.

Visiting Cardiologist, Ryde Hospital, Sydney.

Clinical Associate Professor, Medicine, Concord Clinical School, University of Sydney.

Adjunct Professor, Western Sydney University, New South Wales, Australia.

REFERENCES

Cardiac Failure Explained has been informed by

National Heart Foundation of Australia and Cardiac Society of Australia and New Zealand: Guidelines for the Prevention, Detection, and Management of Heart Failure in Australia 2018

NHFA CSANZ Heart Failure Guidelines Working Group, John J. Atherton, Andrew Sindone, Carmine G. De Pasquale, Andrea Driscoll, Peter S. MacDonald, Ingrid Hopper, Peter M. Kistler, Tom Briffa, James Wong, Walter Abhayaratna, Liza Thomas, Ralph Audehm, Phillip Newton, Joan O'Loughlin, Maree Branagan, Cia Connell.
Heart, Lung and Circulation, October 2018 Volume 27, Issue 10, 1123 - 1208
(https://www.heartlungcirc.org/article/S1443-9506(18)31777-3/fulltext#sec0625)

2017 ACC/AHA/HFSA focused update of the 2013 ACCF/AHA guideline for the management of heart failure: a report of the American College of Cardiology/American Heart Association Task Force on Clinical Practice Guidelines and the Heart Failure Society of America

Clyde W. Yancy, Mariell Jessup, Biykem Bozkurt, Javed Butler, Donald E. Casey Jr, Monica M. Colvin, Mark H. Drazner, Gerasimos S. Filippatos, Gregg C. Fonarow, Michael M. Givertz, Steven M. Hollenberg, JoAnn Lindenfeld, Frederick A. Masoudi, Patrick E. McBride, Pamela N. Peterson, Lynne Warner Stevenson, Cheryl Westlake, Butler J, Casey DE Jr, Colvin MM, Drazner MH, Filippatos GS, Lindenfeld J, Masoudi FA, McBride PE, Peterson PN
(co-published in *Circulation* and the *Journal of Cardiac Failure*)

2016 ESC Guidelines for the diagnosis and treatment of acute and chronic heart failure: The Task Force for the diagnosis and treatment of acute and chronic heart failure of the European Society of Cardiology (ESC) Developed with the special contribution of the Heart Failure Association (HFA) of the ESC

Piotr Ponikowski, Adriaan A Voors, Stefan D Anker, Héctor Bueno, John G F Cleland, Andrew J S Coats, Volkmar Falk, José Ramón González-Juanatey, Veli-Pekka Harjola, Ewa A Jankowska, Mariell Jessup, Cecilia Linde, Petros Nihoyannopoulos, John T Parissis, Burkert Pieske, Jillian P Riley, Giuseppe M C Rosano, Luis M Ruilope, Frank Ruschitzka, Frans H Rutten, Peter van der Meer, ESC Scientific Document Group
European Heart Journal, Volume 37, Issue 27, 14 July 2016, Pages 2129–2200, https://doi.org/10.1093/eurheartj/ehw128
A correction has been published: *European Heart Journal,* Volume 39, Issue 10, 07 March 2018, Page 860, https://doi.org/10.1093/eurheartj/ehw383
A correction has been published: *European Heart Journal,* Volume 39, Issue 14, 07 April 2018, Page 1206, https://doi.org/10.1093/eurheartj/ehx158
Published: 20 May 2016

(released just prior to publication of this book)

CONSENSUS STATEMENT

Universal Definition and Classification of Heart Failure: A Report of the Heart Failure Society of America, Heart Failure Association of the European Society of Cardiology, Japanese Heart Failure Society and Writing Committee of the Universal Definition of Heart Failure

Endorsed by Canadian Heart Failure Society, Heart Failure Association of India, the Cardiac Society of Australia and New Zealand, and the Chinese Heart Failure Association

Biykem Bozkurt, chair; Andrew JS Coats, Hiroyuki Tsutsui, co-chair; Magdy Abdelhamid, Stamatis Adamopoulos, Nancy Albert, Stefan D. Anker,, John Atherton, Michael Böhm, Javed Butler, Mark H. Drazner, G. Michael Felker, Gerasimos Filippatos, Gregg C. Fonarow, Mona Fiuzat, Juan-Esteban Gomez-Mesa, Paul Heidenreich, Teruhiko Imamura, James Januzzi, Ewa A. Jankowska, Prateeti Khazanie, Koichiro Kinugawa, Carolyn S.P. Lam, Yuya Matsue, Marco Metra, Tomohito Ohtani, Massimo Francesco Piepoli, Piotr Ponikowski, Giuseppe M.C. Rosano, Yasushi Sakata, Petar Seferović, Randall C. Starling, John R. Teerlink, Orly Vardeny, Kazuhiro Yamamoto, Clyde Yancy, Jian Zhang, Shelley Zieroth.

Received 2 January 2021, revised 11 January 2021, accepted 13 January 2021.
Journal of Cardiac Failure Vol 27 No 4 2021

For Book Bonuses visit https://drwarrickbishop.com/page/cardiacbookbonus

Never let success get to your head, never let failure get to your heart.

anon.

introduction
A DEFINING CONVERSATION

About 10 years ago, a special patient came into my life. Mary, already in her mid-80s, was notable for her bright blue eyes and her equally bright blue dressing gown. She was also noteworthy for her three daughters who cared enormously for her and had high expectations of me as her cardiologist.

Mary's problem was cardiac failure.

For reasons to do with her heart, she would retain fluid within her body, and that fluid would end up in her lungs (making her short of breath) and in her legs (causing painful swelling). Mary was having a terrible time. She was in and out of hospital almost every four to six weeks, over a couple of years. She would present gasping and swollen and would be admitted. We would 'dry' her out using diuretics, medications to make her pass fluid. She would be in hospital for three to five days and then I would send her home. Each time, I would adjust her medications before discharge and then arrange to see her in the clinic to see how she was traveling. Unfortunately, she was still being hospitalized, very unwell, regularly, until one fateful day.

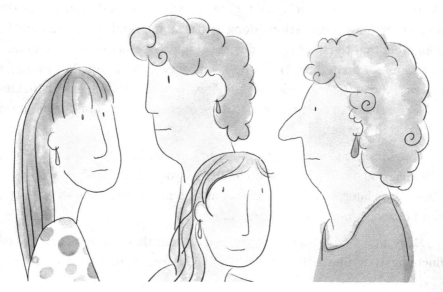

I remember that I was attending Mary on the ward. I was inserting a drip for medication when I asked her for more detail about when the episode had started.

She replied that it was possibly five to six days earlier.

Me: "Did it get gradually worse and worse?"

Mary: "Yes, it did."

Me: "Well, why didn't you come and see me?"

Mary: "Because I was already due to see you in two days, and I didn't want to be a nuisance."

That was a defining conversation. I realized that, with Mary's good understanding of when her health was deteriorating, she potentially could be part of the solution to stop her recurrent admissions.

She was dutifully taking her medications precisely as I had asked her to take them, which is what any doctor would hope a patient would do. However, what was now apparent was that Mary also needed a slightly higher dose of the fluid tablet to drain the fluid away as soon as she recognized there was a problem, such as the beginning of swelling in her legs or the beginning of shortness of breath.

This insight led me to have a long conversation with Mary and with her closely, and eagerly, involved daughters. I was then able to put in place the regular discharge medications along with clear instructions to Mary and her daughters that the fluid tablet dose be doubled immediately should there be any retention of fluid. If the fluid continued to build up, they needed to increase the fluid medication again. They could return to the dose that had been prescribed at the time of discharge once the ankles and the breathing returned to normal.

This simple 'at-home' adjustment, to increase her diuretic therapy dose when she had the first inkling of symptoms, worked incredibly well for Mary. Four weeks later, I saw her in my rooms. No problems. Eight weeks later, I saw her in my rooms again. No problems.

Mary and her daughters had grasped the idea that fluid levels in the body fluctuate from time to time, and when that happened, they had a mechanism to stop it spiraling out of control. That simple intervention kept Mary out of hospital for more than 18 months, compared to her history of hospital admission every four-to-six weeks.

This experience with Mary started me on a different journey with cardiac failure. It showed me how important it is to engage the patient and look at that individual's situation from a day-to-day basis, knowing that the patient is the person best placed to understand his/her body and particular needs. I realized that caring for cardiac failure at home, where possible, was better than caring for it in the clinic and definitely better than in the hospital. Of course, those adjustments at home do not always work. However, as Mary's example highlights, and as I have found subsequently for many of my patients, they can be a great help.

cardiac failure

Cardiac failure, or heart failure, is a weighty illness in today's society. The condition affects about one in 10 people aged 75 years or older. It is rapidly becoming one of the biggest medical challenges and usurps coronary artery disease as the most significant heart-related condition in the western world. Suffered by millions of people, cardiac failure impacts individuals, families, and communities. Due to the high cost of treatment and care, it also has a significant bearing on economies, accounting for about 10 percent of the total healthcare budget in western countries. Not only is it a significant condition, it is also a complicated one.

Cardiac failure occurs when the heart does not pump as well as it should.

The heart is the pump that supplies blood to all the organs of the body. If the heart is not functioning properly, the circulation will inevitably be compromised and this will adversely affect any number of the body's organs.

One of the most common cardiac failure presentations is **shortness of breath**, often occurring during exercise. However, shortness of breath can also occur at rest and may even happen while the patient is asleep, waking up the person who is gasping for air. Cardiac failure may also be associated with **swelling** because of fluid retention. Importantly, though, because the heart supplies blood to every organ in the body, people suffering cardiac failure may also present with symptoms that involve fatigue, including muscle fatigue, an inability to undertake daily living activities, depression, and memory impairment. Sometimes, in severe cases, the liver becomes dysfunctional. Blood can flow back from the heart through the inferior vena cava to the liver, leading to swelling and congestion in that organ. A swollen and congested liver doesn't function well, so liver impairment, and even failure, can ensue.

The heart and the liver are near each other in the body.

compromised circulation

To explain the responses of the body to a heart that is not working correctly, let's go back several million years, to our ancestors. Imagine that a sabretooth tiger has bitten an ancestor. The ancestor is bleeding and has lost a lot of blood but not enough to die. His circulation is compromised; his body has sensors or **receptors** which continuously assess the efficiency and adequacy of the body's circulation. These receptors are in the **heart**, in the body's **major blood vessels** (the carotid arteries and the aorta), and also in the **kidneys**. When they sense a lack of blood volume in the circulation, the receptors trigger responses, principally through the kidneys, to increase blood pressure and retain fluid.

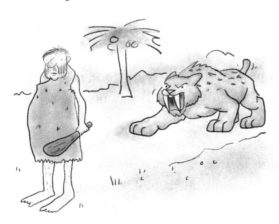

Now, this is a fantastic mechanism if a sabretooth tiger has just bitten you, as you want your body in a mode where it's maintaining blood pressure and storing fluid to replenish the circulation, thus ensuring the blood flows properly to all the vital organs.

Fast-forward two million years.

Our bodies still retain the same evolutionary receptors and responses. Let's imagine now that, for whatever reason, the heart stops working as well as it should, meaning that there is a degree of cardiac failure, which compromises the circulation. Those receptors that have worked well in humans for millions of years realize that there is a problem. The receptors – in the heart, blood vessels and kidneys – notice a problem with the circulation that registers as if there is not enough blood volume in the circulation. Their response, as it has been across the millennia, is to start to maintain blood pressure and retain fluid. The problem is that now they are reacting in a closed circuit (there is no fluid or blood loss from the body as there was with the sabretooth tiger) and there is nowhere for the extra fluid to go; it has to build up in the body. As fluid can collect in the lungs, and in the periphery of the body, such as the legs, this contributes to the shortness of breath and the swelling of feet and legs, as evidenced in cardiac failure. This physiological preservation response that worked particularly well in an entirely different setting for our ancestors, now works poorly.

Heart failure, in essence, is the heart no longer pumping effectively. This becomes a complex mix of

- **a sick heart,**
- **maladapted responses to the impaired circulation and**
- **fluid retention that further strains the heart, starting a downward spiral.**

Potentially, every organ of the body can be impacted.

Several conditions underpin heart failure and there are a number of possible outcomes for the patient.

The following pages tease out for you the most relevant information about how we understand the condition, how we diagnose it, what we can do to treat it, and how the patient can competently live with it.

Did you know that responding to increased thirst is a means of rebuilding and replenishing the body's fluid volume?

- Some conditions that lead to heart failure can be reversed, improving the symptoms of heart failure and helping the patient live longer. Always though, "the best way to manage heart failure is to prevent it"[1].

- In one type of heart failure, the heart can appear to pump normally.

- Heart failure can manifest differently in men and women.

- Heart disease is the number one killer of women[2]; deadlier than all forms of cancer combined. Cardiac failure is today's foremost heart disease.

- Controlling blood pressure and maintaining a healthy weight are two of the most important things a person can do to reduce the risk of developing heart failure.

- Yoga and exercise are good for heart failure patients.

- Heart failure can run in families.

---

[1]   *How to Manage Heart Failure: New Guidelines 2018; Garry L.R. Jennings MD, FRACP, Cia Connell B Pharm, M Clinic Pharm; Heart, Lung and Circulation (2018) 27, 1267-1269*

[2]   *Heart disease is the leading cause of death for women in the United States, killing 299,578 women in 2017, or about 1 in every 5 female deaths*
https://www.cdc.gov/heartdisease/women.htm

Heart disease is the number one killer of Australian women, killing three times as many women as breast cancer. An Australian woman dies from heart disease every hour and 50 women suffer a heart attack every day. More than 48,000 women are treated in hospital for heart disease every year.

https://www.hri.org.au/health/learn/cardiovascular-disease/women-and-heart-disease

And now for the absorbing details.

THE HEART
SOME BASIC UNDERSTANDINGS

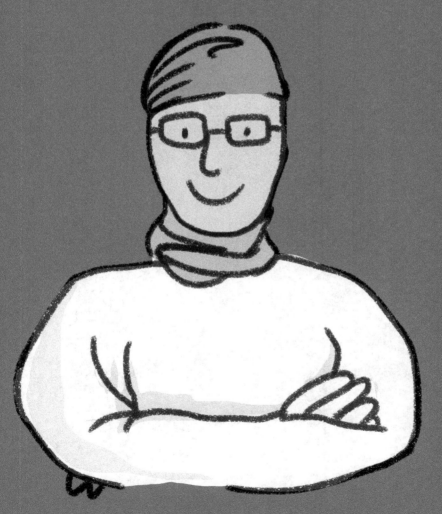

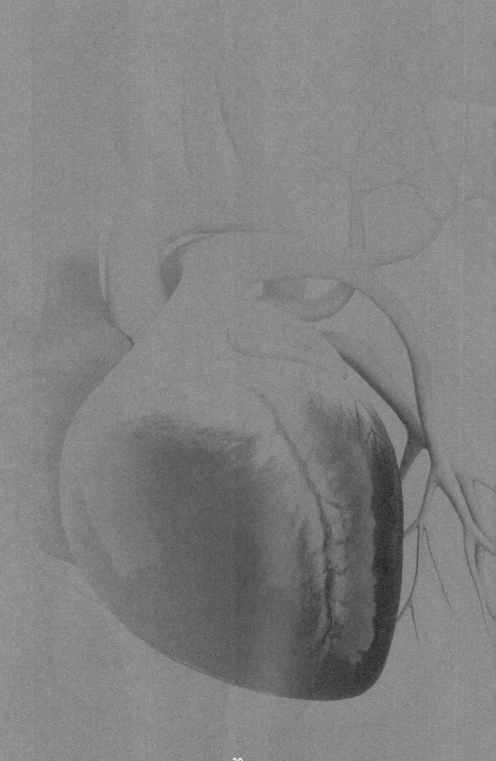

chapter 1
A HIGH-FUNCTIONING ENGINE

The interchangeable terms, heart failure (HF), cardiac failure (CF) and congestive cardiac failure (CCF), can be quite overwhelming for people if they ever think about them. Although a functioning heart is critical for human life, your heart beats away in your chest doing its thing until something appears to go wrong: it doesn't perform as well as expected; becomes deficient or insufficient; stops working properly. Our most common, almost immediate, response when something goes wrong with the heart is to think 'heart attack' and yet there are several other severe conditions that affect this life-sustaining organ. Heart failure is one, meaning the muscle or pumping chamber of the heart is affected. Others include arrhythmias, when the electrical system is at fault, and coronary artery disease (CAD), which involves the arteries that supply blood to the heart.

Before we delve further into the specifics of cardiac failure, let's look at what makes the heart 'tick' as it was designed to work.

....

CARDIOVASCULAR DISEASE (CVD) *is the general term for conditions affecting the heart or blood vessels and includes coronary heart disease, angina, heart attack, congenital heart disease, stroke and vascular dementia. In the UNITED STATES, one person dies every 37 seconds from cardiovascular disease. About 647,000 Americans die from heart disease every year. Coronary artery disease (CAD) is the most common manifestation of cardiovascular disease, killing 365,914 people in the USA in 2017. In AUSTRALIA, heart disease accounted for 18,590 deaths in 2017. Although heart disease deaths have decreased by 22 percent in the past decade, in 2017, 51 Australians died from heart disease each day, or a death every 28 minutes. In the UNITED KINGDOM, CVD affects about seven million people or over 10 percent of the population and is a significant cause of disability and death.*

....

a healthy heart

The heart is primarily a large muscle that pumps blood through our bodies so that the blood supplies nutrients and oxygen to all parts of the body and removes waste such as carbon dioxide. A well-functioning heart contracts rhythmically, pumping blood to the body roughly **100,000 times a day**, which is about 35 million times a year and over three billion times in a lifetime!

Wow! That's a lot of work!

The heart can be likened to a car engine, with compression chambers and valves, an electrical system and fuel lines.

As a car engine has an **electrical system** for timing, so does the heart. The electrical system in the heart ensures synchronicity and coordinated contraction throughout the heart. It also allows for acceleration and deceleration of the heart as a pump.

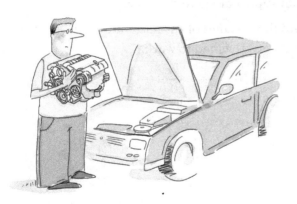

The car has **pistons and valves;** its engine block is the part that generates the power. In the heart, the pistons are the compression chambers, the main one being the left ventricle, while several valves stop the blood flowing back from where it has been pumped.

The car engine also requires a fuel line to supply the engine block. In the human heart, the coronary arteries are **fuel lines** that provide the lifeblood to the engine block.

Within the heart's structure, there are two chambers on the right-hand side and two chambers on the left-hand side so that on each side of the heart there is a **pre-pumping chamber, the atrium**, and the **main pumping chamber, the ventricle**.

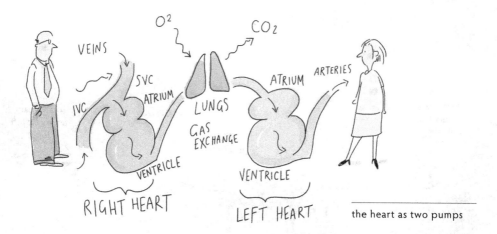

the heart as two pumps

This means the heart has **two pumps**, one which accepts the blood back from the body and then pumps it to the lungs for carbon dioxide/oxygen exchange, and a second pump which receives the blood from the lungs and then drives it around the body. These are the 'right heart' and the 'left heart', respectively. The sides pump together with each atrium contracting marginally ahead of its ventricle.

Blood flows from the body to the heart through the veins, collecting into two major veins called the **superior vena cava** (SVC) ① *(refer to diagram next page)* and the **inferior vena cava** (IVC) ① which drain into the right side of the heart. This oxygen-poor, dark purple, carbon dioxide-rich blood arrives in the **right atrium** ② where it receives a gentle pump through the **tricuspid** valve, a one-way valve, into the **right ventricle** ③. The ventricle then pumps the blood through another one-way valve, the **pulmonary** valve, into the **lungs,** via the **pulmonary artery** ④⑤.

Within the lungs, gas exchange occurs; the air we breathe in provides oxygen and the breath we exhale carries away carbon dioxide. The blood becomes replenished with fresh oxygen for use by the body.

Bright red, oxygen-rich arterial blood then flows from the lungs through the **four pulmonary veins** ⑥ to the **left atrium** ⑦. The left atrium gives a gentle pump and the blood passes through the **mitral** valve, another one-way valve, into the **left ventricle** ⑧. The left ventricle then contracts, squeezing blood through the **aortic** valve, another one-way valve, into the main artery of the body, the **aorta** ⑨⑩, to begin its journey around the body. **The left ventricle is the main pumping chamber of the heart.**

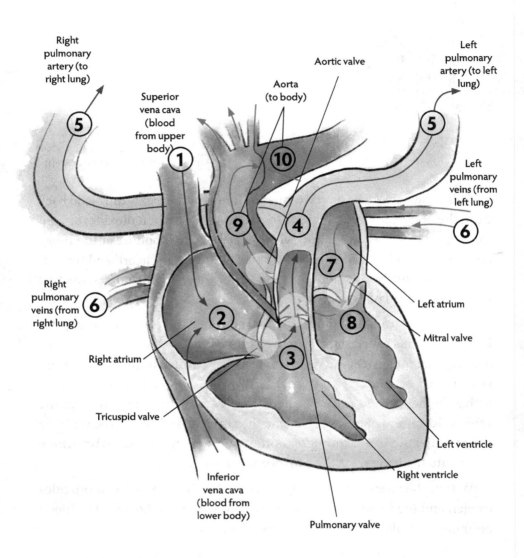

Right pulmonary artery (to right lung)

5

Superior vena cava (blood from upper body)

1

Aortic valve

Aorta (to body)

10

Left pulmonary artery (to left lung)

5

Left pulmonary veins (from left lung)

9 **4**

6

Right pulmonary veins (from right lung)

6

2

7

3

8

Left atrium

Mitral valve

Right atrium

Tricuspid valve

Left ventricle

Inferior vena cava (blood from lower body)

Right ventricle

Pulmonary valve

the pathway of blood flow through the heart

the components of the heart

the fuel lines – the coronary arteries

The **coronary arteries** arise from the aorta as it comes from the left ventricle. These are the fuel lines of the heart engine and they are the first branches in the **circulatory system.**

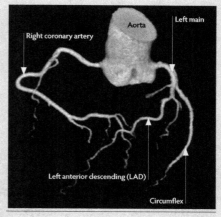

The coronary tree as seen on cardiac CT imaging.

If we think of the arteries as the fuel lines supplying the cylinders of the car, this system consists of the **left main coronary artery** and the **right coronary artery**. Within one centimeter the **left main coronary artery** divides into two arteries:

- the **left anterior descending artery** which provides blood to the anterior surface of the heart, which is the surface nearest the chest wall, and

- the **circumflex artery** which supplies blood to the back of the heart, which is the surface of the heart nearest the spine.

The **right coronary artery** supplies the inferior surface of the heart, which is the surface that is nearest the diaphragm.

The terms 'right dominant' or 'left dominant' are used in reference to the artery that supplies blood to the bulk of the inferior surface of the heart (the surface nearest the diaphragm). This is usually from the right coronary artery and, therefore, termed 'right dominant'. Sometimes, however, the right coronary artery is smaller and the circumflex artery (the one that branches off the left main coronary artery) is bigger, or 'dominant'. When the left coronary artery supplies the majority of the inferior surface of the heart, it is called 'left dominant'. Size becomes significant in terms of the amount of the heart that may be affected by a blockage of the artery, the dominant artery providing blood to a larger territory.

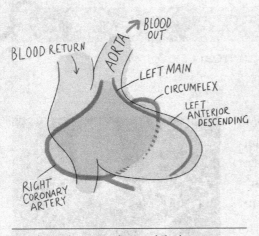

blood vessels wrapped around the heart

Most often, the **left anterior descending artery** is the largest and most important of the three main coronary arteries. It can be 12 to 14 cm long while only two to five millimeters in diameter. This dimension is a little thicker than a pen refill, yet its blockage can be disastrous. A dominant right coronary artery can be approximately the same size and a non-dominant circumflex can be six to eight centimeters long and 1.5 to three millimeters in diameter.

The major arteries are comprised of fewer than 35 cm in total length and fewer than five millimeters in diameter at their largest. This is a very vulnerable system.

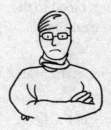

It doesn't matter in which Western country you live, nor does it much matter your ethnic group or sex, heart disease remains the leading cause of death. PLEASE! PLEASE! PLEASE!
Always seek immediate medical attention should you be affected by chest pain or unexplained shortness of breath.

the electrical system

A healthy heart is a highly efficient pump coordinated by its electrical system. The atria and ventricles work together, alternately contracting and relaxing, to pump blood through the heart and into the body. Electrical impulses trigger the heartbeat.

Typically, the contractions of the atria are set off by the heart's natural pacemaker, a small area of the heart called the **sinoatrial (SA) node,** located in the top of the right atrium. The SA node is where the electrical activity 'beats the drum' to which the rest of the heart 'marches'.

26

Electrical impulses travel rapidly throughout the atria, somewhat like a Mexican wave, causing the muscle fibers to contract, squeezing blood into the ventricles. To reach the ventricles, these electrical impulses pass through the **atrioventricular** (AV) node, a cluster of cells in the center of the heart, between the atria and the ventricles.

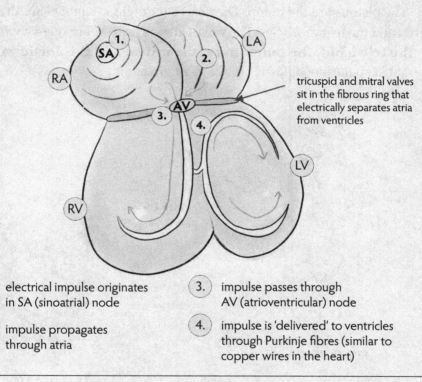

tricuspid and mitral valves sit in the fibrous ring that electrically separates atria from ventricles

1. electrical impulse originates in SA (sinoatrial) node

2. impulse propagates through atria

3. impulse passes through AV (atrioventricular) node

4. impulse is 'delivered' to ventricles through Purkinje fibres (similar to copper wires in the heart)

the electrical system

This node acts as a gatekeeper. Passing through this node slows the electrical impulses before they enter the ventricles, thus giving the atria time to contract before the ventricles then contract. Once in the ventricles, specialized cells, called Purkinje Fibers, carry the electrical impulse. The Purkinje fibers act like wires delivering the signal to the apex of the heart and ensure that blood is expelled from the furthest point first.

This normal heart rhythm is known as **sinus rhythm** because it is controlled by the sinoatrial, or sinus, node. In a healthy heart, this beating is synchronistic and smooth. Visualize, if you can, a squid moving through the water. Synchronous. Coordinated. Smooth. When this synchronicity breaks down, **heart arrhythmias** occur such as atrial fibrillation, atrial or ventricular ectopic beats, atrial flutter, supra-ventricular tachycardia, ventricular tachycardia, and ventricular fibrillation.

the pistons and valves

The pistons are the pump. The heart's pumping chambers are the two atria and the two ventricles. The valves are the heart's four one-way valves **– the tricuspid, the pulmonary, the mitral and the aortic valves** – that keep the blood flowing in the right direction.

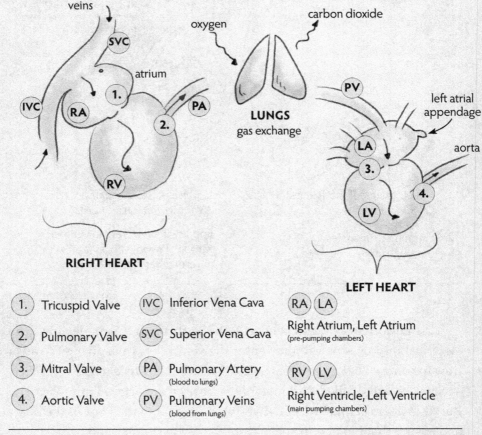

1.	Tricuspid Valve	IVC	Inferior Vena Cava	RA LA
2.	Pulmonary Valve	SVC	Superior Vena Cava	Right Atrium, Left Atrium (pre-pumping chambers)
3.	Mitral Valve	PA	Pulmonary Artery (blood to lungs)	RV LV
4.	Aortic Valve	PV	Pulmonary Veins (blood from lungs)	Right Ventricle, Left Ventricle (main pumping chambers)

the valves within the heart

the blood

Another significant element in this system is the fuel – the blood. Blood contains red cells which are carriers of **hemoglobin**, the oxygen-carrying substance that transports oxygen to the body's tissues. A good supply of oxygen is critical for the proper functioning of the heart and other body organs. **Platelets** are the other essential component of the blood. As platelets stop us bleeding, for example, when we cut ourselves, damage within the vascular system needs these small particles to form clots (thrombi). The blood also carries **nutrients** and **fats** such as cholesterol.

the circulation

Finally, there is the **carrier** of the fuel to the body, the circulation. Keeping in mind the above sections of the heart, imagine the circulation as a closed loop, like a tire inner tube containing fluid that passes around the tube in a single direction.

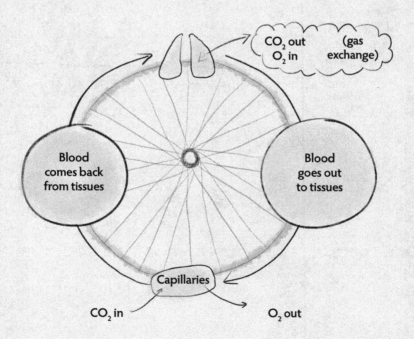

Moving clockwise from the lungs at 12 o'clock, the fluid, the oxygenated blood, passes through the heart's left atrium and then left ventricle, goes into the body to the organs where it provides oxygen and nutrients to the tissues. The blood, having passed through the capillaries, then collects in the veins which join into two major veins, the superior vena cava (SVC, which drains the top of the body) and the inferior vena cava (IVC, which drains the lower section of the body). The blood passes into the right atrium and then right ventricle and circulates back into the lungs, and the cycle repeats itself.

As the lungs and the heart are within the thorax, **breathing** also has an impact on return blood flow. *(We will examine the circulation more thoroughly in the next chapter.)*

The circulatory system is one of three places within the body where we find fluid. The other places are <u>within</u> *cells (intracellular fluid that includes all fluid enclosed in cells by their walls or membranes) and* <u>between</u> *cells (the extracellular fluid). When fluid builds up in a person's feet, the fluid has moved out of the blood vessels and into the surrounding tissues. It is extracellular.*

Blood vessel (circulation)

Cells

Tissue

Intracellular

Extracellular

Tissue

cascade of consequences

When a person suffers cardiac failure because the heart is not pumping enough blood around the body, a cascade of consequences results in calamity for the person whose heart is not working correctly.

The body, not receiving enough blood, turns on a **neurohumoral** response (*neuro*, nerves; *humoral*, messengers within the blood), the 'fight' or 'flight' response.

If you have ever been frightened, you will have experienced your heart racing.

The lack of cardiac output, which registers as a lack of blood volume by organs within the body, triggers the receptors in the major blood vessels and kidneys and the neurohumoral response says,

> "Wow! We've lost blood. We need to preserve what we can. We need to keep the blood pressure up and get the blood volume back."

This response signals to the body to constrict blood vessels in the periphery (arms and legs) so that the blood pressure to the vital organs remains elevated and to retain fluid to replenish what it perceives to be lost fluid from bleeding out.

These responses feed back to the heart which becomes even more loaded and inflamed (a localized cellular response to trauma which may cause its own detrimental effect). The body, now responding to a heart that's not working properly, experiences

- **vasoconstriction,** or increased tension in the blood vessels **to keep up the blood pressure;**

- **fluid retention to increase blood volume;**

- a **racing** and

- **inflamed** heart

all of which load the heart even further, which stimulates the neurohumoral response into 'thinking' the situation is getting worse, and so the vicious cycle continues and compounds.

(We will examine the autonomic nervous system more thoroughly in chapter 4 and also look at the responses and how we may attempt to avert them to protect the heart in the long-term.)

Additionally, other medical conditions can feed into this deteriorating health scenario, resulting in further consequences. **Age, coronary artery disease** and **atrial fibrillation** are common **associations** of cardiac failure.

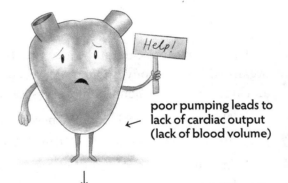

Associations of cardiac failure include:
- age
- coronary artery disease
- atrial fibrillation

poor pumping leads to lack of cardiac output (lack of blood volume)

↓

neurohumoral response
triggered by receptors in major blood vessels and kidneys
(needs to preserve what it can)

↓   ↓   ↓

peripheral
vasocontriction
blood pressure up

racing
heart

fluid retention
congestion in the lungs
shortness of breath
swelling in the legs

↘   ↓   ↙

receptors think there is a problem
vicious cycle repeats, compounds situation

Consequences include:
- general fatigue
- skeletal muscle fatigue
- iron depletion
- renal dysfunction
- depression
- poor sleep, altered memory, confusion
- heart scarring

a sick heart

Consequences of cardiac failure lead to

general fatigue	poor sleep, not feeling 'right', depressed mood, decreased exercise capacity and the effort to overcome shortness of breath all contribute to a sense of general fatigue
skeletal muscle fatigue	lack of blood flow means the muscles do not receive the blood they need and that leads to muscle fatigue
iron depletion	cardiac failure changes proteins that are available for iron absorption. When the body stops absorbing iron efficiently, not enough is available for heart function and iron levels drop. At worst the patient can develop **anemia** which aggravates the situation.
renal dysfunction	the kidneys suffer because they need good blood flow to maintain good filtration
depression	the nature of the symptoms, their impact on daily living, uncertainty, and even side-effects of medications can drag down the individual
poor sleep	as the heart fails to work during the day, it also fails to work during the night. Patients can have disturbed sleep leading to altered memory and confusion.
scarring	stress and strain on the heart in an environment of an activated 'flight or fight' response will generate inflammation in the heart tissues and subsequent micro scarring.

This is a terrible cycle of the heart not working correctly, with the body driving responses that plummet cardiac failure into a downward spiral.

A functioning heart is like a well-oiled engine, working smoothly and efficiently with the help of fuel lines, the engine block and its electrical circuit to ensure that it works as expected.

When a heart does not work properly (cardiac failure)

- neurohumoral response, 'fight or flight' response, drives
  - increased blood pressure
  - fluid retention
  - increased heart rate
  - inflammation

and then the whole cycle feeds back on itself.

Cardiac failure associations include, most commonly,

- age
- coronary artery disease
- atrial fibrillation.

Cardiac failure consequences include

- skeletal muscle fatigue
- iron depletion
- renal dysfunction
- poor sleep

and their numerous implications.

Before getting down to the nitty-gritty of cardiac failure, several concepts are critical to understanding how the body works and reacts under this pressure.

chapter 2
BODY PUMPS, PIPES AND REGULATORS

We need to discuss several other elements before moving on. Over the next three chapters, we will learn about

- how well the heart pumps and how that is measured (ejection fraction) and

- blood flow (circulation) [chapter 2],

- the kidneys and

- the lungs [chapter 3], and

- the systems that come into play when the body's fluid balance becomes challenged,

  - the 'fight or flight' response (autonomic nervous system),

  - the blood pressure and salt balancing (renin-angiotensin-aldosterone) system

  - the body's own heart tonics (natriuretic peptide system) [chapter 4].

I know this sounds a bit intense, but, please, hang in with me. These are important concepts to understand for coming to grips with heart failure and how we treat it. I hope to explain them in simple terms.

ejection fraction

A critical indicator of how well the heart is working is the **ejection fraction (EF)**, the term used in association with the **left ventricle**, the main pumping chamber of the heart. The left ventricle (LV) is muscular and is shaped like the end of a bullet. It is also hollow, so that when the blood flows in, the LV relaxes and fills and, as the LV contracts, it pushes the

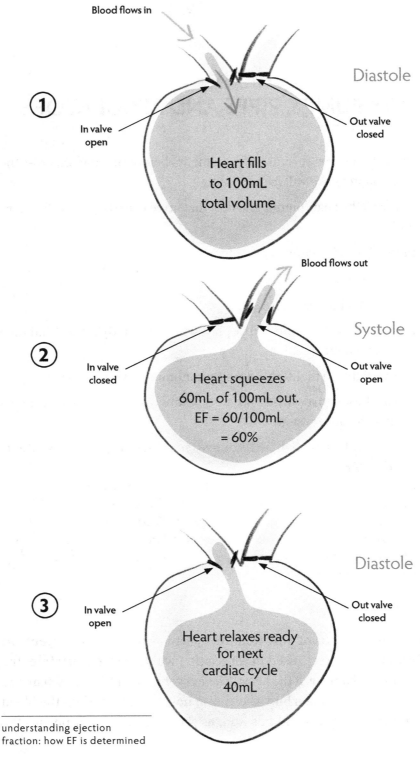

Blood flows in

Diastole

(1)

In valve
open

Out valve
closed

Heart fills
to 100mL
total volume

Blood flows out

Systole

(2)

In valve
closed

Out valve
open

Heart squeezes
60mL of 100mL out.
EF = 60/100mL
= 60%

Diastole

(3)

In valve
open

Out valve
closed

Heart relaxes ready
for next
cardiac cycle
40mL

understanding ejection
fraction: how EF is determined

blood out into the body. When the blood flows in and the heart is resting, it is called **diastole**; when the heart contracts, it is called **systole**.

EF refers to the amount of blood ejected from the left ventricle with each heartbeat, expressed as a percentage of the total volume of blood contained within the left ventricle.

What is significant about the EF is that the chamber does not squeeze down or contract entirely and so it **does not empty completely, even for a normal heartbeat in a healthy heart.** The ejection fraction would be 100 percent if the chamber expelled every drop. However, that is not the case. A healthy left ventricle squeezes out only a proportion of the blood, about 60 percent.

In a healthy heart, this percentage will increase with exercise.

So nominally, if the heart holds 100mL, the contraction expels about 60mL, giving an ejection fraction of 60 percent. The normal range is between 55 and 65 percent.

It is important to understand what the ejection fraction is a percentage of – and it is not 100 percent. Confusion often arises because people automatically think 100 percent must be normal. One hundred percent would occur if the LV expelled all the blood it contained in one beat, yet a healthy heart expels only 55 to 65 percent of the blood. So as an example, an EF 40 percent is not a reduction of 60 percent of the normal. It is a reduction of function of $1-40/60 = 1-0.66 = 0.33$ which is one third.

Although an EF of 40 percent is not ideal, it is a 30 percent reduction of the standard 60 percent EF, and poses a less confronting situation than 40 percent of 100 percent which would give a decline in function of 60 percent!

A patient with an EF of

- **less than 50 percent** classifies as having a **reduced** EF (HFrEF) or **systolic** failure (the heart **does not contract** properly, and so it doesn't push out as much blood as it should);

- **50 percent or higher** classifies as having a **preserved** EF (HFpEF) or **diastolic** failure (the heart contracts normally but **fails to relax,** limiting the LV's refilling ability; a consequence of a stiff or thickened heart muscle);

The ejection fraction is most commonly measured using ultrasound, or an **echocardiogram**, of the heart. EF can also be measured using:

- nuclear medicine techniques,

- magnetic resonance imaging,

- CT scanning of the heart, and

- direct injection of contrast into the heart.

When it comes to treatment, each of the major EFs has its peculiarities. HFrEF tends to respond to treatment while HFpEF, which is more prevalent in the Western world, has a poorer response. Of note, the incidence of HFpEF is rising due to the increasing rates of its co-morbidities including age, blood pressure, obesity and diabetes.

Discussions about blood pressure use the terms diastole and systole, relating to the two figures recorded. The top figure is the systolic blood pressure and is the highest pressure when the heart is pumping, while diastolic blood pressure, the number recorded underneath, is the pressure in the circulation system when the heart is resting.

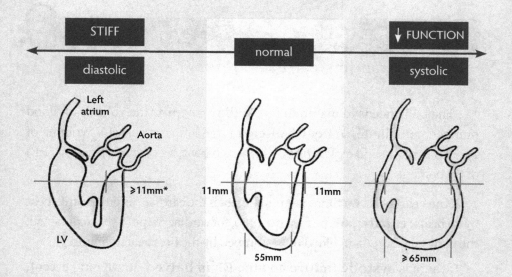

HFpEF	normal heart	HFrEF
EF 50% +	EF about 60%	EF - 50%
diastolic		systolic
contracts ok BUT fails to relax = stiff heart (limits the LV to fill to capacity)		fails to contract properly
heart is normal size	heart is normal size	heart is dilated *(see next page)*
very hard to treat; does not respond well to current therapies		responds well to current therapies
incidence rising due to co-morbidities such as age, hypertension, obesity, diabetes		
most common form of heart failure in Western societies		

ejection fraction

understanding cardiac output

The body needs to maintain its **cardiac output** (the volume of blood pumped per minute). A **healthy heart** has a left ventricle (LV) volume of 100mL of blood and expels 60mL with each beat, an ejection fraction (EF) of 60 percent.

If the heart beats 60 times per minute, then the cardiac output (60mL/beat by 60 beats) **equals 3.6L per minute**. So, for cardiac output to be maintained, the body 'needs' 3.6L of blood to be pumped by the heart each minute.

If there is **systolic failure** and the **EF is halved**, to say 30 percent, then, in order to maintain the same cardiac output, the **heart rate needs to double.** Cardiac output compared to a normal heart is now 30mL (30% EF, was 60% EF) multiplied by 120 beats (was 60 bpm) = 3.6L/minute.

If there is systolic failure and the EF is halved to 30 percent **but the heart rate doesn't increase** then

cardiac output = 3.6L = 30% of new LV volume by 60 bpm

3.6L ÷ 60 bpm = 30% of new LV volume

3.6L ÷ 60×100/30 = new LV volume = 200mL

→ dilated cardiomyopathy

Both instances of systolic failure occur in response to decreased EF, resulting in increased heart rate or increased left ventricle volume.

	normal	↓EF LV size stays the same	↓EF heart rate stays the same
EF	60%	30%	30%
LV volume	100 mL	100 mL	200 mL
blood expelled each beat stroke volume (SV)	EF x LV volume 60% x 100 mL = 60 mL	EF x LV volume 30% x 100 mL = 30mL	EF x LV volume 30% x 200 mL = 60mL
beats per minute (bpm)	60 bpm	120 bpm	60 bpm
cardiac output	SV x bpm 60 mL x 60 bpm = 3.6 L/minute	SV x bpm 30 mL x 120 bpm = 3.6 L/minute	SV x bpm 60 mL x 60 bpm = 3.6 L/minute

understanding cardiac output

the circle of circulation

One of the most important jobs of the circulatory system is to take oxygen from the air to the body's tissues and dispel the waste product, carbon dioxide. In cardiac failure, the lungs are one of the circulation's most significant components.

Let's drill down a little further as we ask the questions:

- How does the blood keep going around the body?

- Why is this important in medical considerations of the heart?

Remember, our inner tube contains a pump and several one-way valves? The heart is the pump and the one-way valves ensure the flow keeps going in the right direction, that is, clockwise. So, where does the heart fit within this flow?

journey

Let's start again at the lungs where the carbon dioxide/oxygen gas exchange takes place.

Bright red, oxygen-rich blood flows from the lungs through the four pulmonary veins to the left atrium of the heart. In the left atrium, the blood gets a gentle pump that moves it through the one-way mitral valve into the left ventricle, which is the primary pumping chamber. The blood passes through

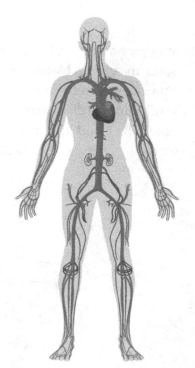

Circulatory System

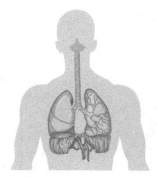

Respiratory System

The circulatory and respiratory systems work together to move blood and oxygen/carbon dioxide throughout the body. Breath containing the oxygen (breath in) and carbon dioxide (breath out) moves in and out of the lungs through the trachea, bronchi and bronchioles. Blood moves in an out of the lungs, where the gas exchange occurs, through the pulmonary arteries and veins that connect the lungs with the heart.

41

another one-way valve, the aortic valve, so that it can only flow into the aorta, the biggest blood vessel coming out of the heart. The blood's journey continues from the aorta into the organs of the body and then through smaller and smaller arteries until it reaches the capillary bed of those organs. When the blood has passed through the capillary bed, it then collects in increasingly more prominent veins as it makes its way back to the heart.

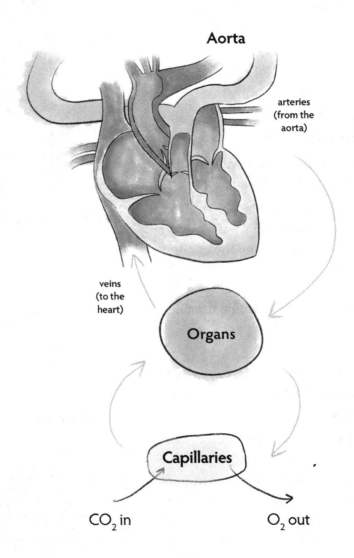

journey of the blood

The veins collect together until they become two major inlets into the right atrium of the heart. The superior vena cava (SVC) collects the blood draining from above

Imagine a mirror image - the arteries get smaller and smaller, and the veins get bigger and bigger.

the heart and the inferior vena cava (IVC) collects the blood flowing from below the heart. This by-now dark purple, carbon dioxide-rich, oxygen-poor blood, accumulates in the right atrium. It gets a gentle pump and another one-way valve, the tricuspid valve, ensures that it continues to flow in a clockwise direction into the right ventricle. From there, the blood passes through the pulmonary artery into the lungs. The carbon dioxide/oxygen gas exchange occurs and the blood then runs passively through the four pulmonary veins into the left atrium, and the journey continues.

The heart beats, on average, about 100,000 times per day, pumping five or six quarts of blood each minute, or about 2000 gallons per day. It is a lot of blood and a lot of work!

organs

Now, let's add some organs into the journey as we continue to build the complexity of the system.

As the blood leaves the heart, it moves into the aorta, which divides into arteries that supply the major organs within the body. The first blood vessels that come off the aorta supply the **heart** itself, so that the heart supplies the blood that drives the muscle that runs the heart, the myocardium (*myo*, muscle; *cardium*, of the heart), the muscular middle layer of the wall of the heart.

After the heart, the next major organ supplied by blood traveling through the circulatory system is the **brain**. Nearly 25 percent of the blood circulating around the body goes to the brain, supplied by the carotid and vertebral arteries.

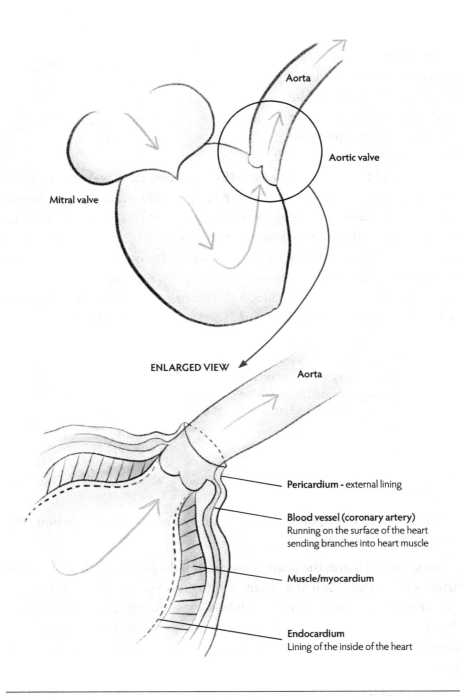

Aorta

Aortic valve

Mitral valve

ENLARGED VIEW

Aorta

Pericardium - external lining

Blood vessel (coronary artery)
Running on the surface of the heart
sending branches into heart muscle

Muscle/myocardium

Endocardium
Lining of the inside of the heart

Layers of the heart: The heart wall is made up of three layers: the outer layer is the **pericardium** (fibrous tissues that form a protective sac that holds the heart together), the middle layer is the **myocardium** (middle layer of thick muscle, the cardiac muscle that drives the cardiac cycle and the first part of the body to receive the oxygen-rich blood) and the inner layer, the **endocardium** (a thin layer of epithelial cells that line the cavities and the valves).

A healthy heart at rest pumps about four liters of blood per minute around the body. The brain requires about one liter of that blood to supply it with the oxygen and nutrients it needs to function well and to take away carbon dioxide and other waste materials.

The **kidneys** need nearly 25 percent as they busily clean the blood, filtering out impurities and making urine. The **gut** gets blood; the amount varies depending on circumstances such as if you have recently had a meal. **Muscles** also receive blood, the amount of which depends on circumstances such as if you are at rest or exercising.

These organs take the blood through smaller and smaller arteries (arterioles) until they become the very small and very fine blood vessels, the capillaries. They are so fine they allow the exchange of

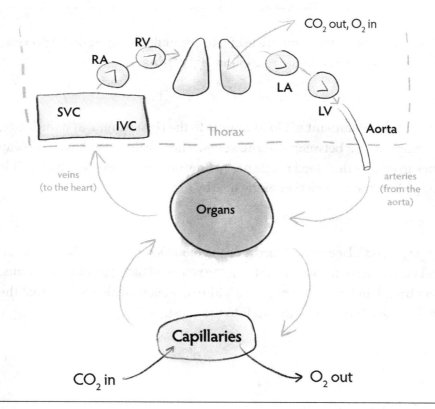

circle of circulation

oxygen and carbon dioxide through their membranes. Although nutrients and other products within the blood also move back and forth, for ease, our focus is the gas exchange. As the blood continues its journey, the capillaries form veins and the veins form the IVC or the SVC, depending on the part of the body from which the blood comes.

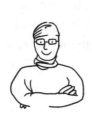

Another way of thinking about the circulation system is to compare it to an irrigation system. The main pump is the heart and the main outlet pipe is the aorta. From there, the water (blood) travels through a variety of pipes (arteries) to different fields (organs and muscles). Instead of the water soaking into the ground, the blood is returned to the main pump via the veins, initially small and getting larger, before closing the loop of reticulation or circulation.

Two other considerations are useful to our understanding of the process, the role of **muscles** and the role of our **breathing**.

massaging the blood back to the heart

A significant amount of blood returns to the right atrium, and the lungs, via veins that lie between the **muscles**. These veins also have one-way valves to ensure the blood continues to flow in a clockwise direction as it is 'pumped' by the contraction of the nearby muscle.

sucking the blood back to the heart

The person's **breathing** also aids the blood's return. The thorax, or the chest cavity, helps the venous return, the return of blood through the veins. Every breath in lowers the pressure within the chest, which means that the blood outside the chest is drawn into the chest.

Ejection fraction (EF) indicates how well the left ventricle (LV) is working

- how well the heart contracts with each beat
- expressed as a percentage of the total volume of blood in the LV before contraction begins
  - systolic (contracting)
    - bad heart with 50 percent or lower – reduced – systolic failure
  - diastolic (resting)
    - bad heart with 50 percent or higher – preserved – diastolic failure

Circulation

- takes oxygen from the lungs to the body's tissues via the arteries, arterioles and capillaries
- moves carbon dioxide to the lungs for the gas exchange via veins
- important components (moving from the lungs)
  - lungs (carbon dioxide/oxygen exchange)
  - four pulmonary veins
  - left atrium
  - mitral valve
  - left ventricle (main pumping chamber)
  - aortic valve
  - aorta, major arteries

(continued next page)

- organs
  - heart
  - brain
  - kidneys
  - gut
    - smaller and smaller arteries within the organs
    - capillary bed
    - bigger and bigger veins
- major veins
- IVC or SVC
- right atrium
- tricuspid valve
- right ventricle
- pulmonary artery
- lungs (carbon dioxide/oxygen exchange)
- other elements
  - muscles
  - breath

We learn about two crucial 'neighbors' of the heart, the renal system and the lungs, in the next chapter.

chapter 3
CLOSE NEIGHBORS

As we expand our understanding of the complexities involved with cardiac failure, it is essential to understand the workings of two close 'neighbors' to the heart, the kidneys and the lungs.

the kidneys

The body has two 'treatment plants', the bean-shaped kidneys, which are the primary organs of the body's renal system. Each is about the size of a fist, with one on each side of the spine below the rib-cage in the middle of the back. They are a "very complex, environmentally friendly, waste disposal system (that sorts) non-recyclable waste from recyclable waste, 24 hours a day, seven days a week, while also cleaning your blood"[3]. While a person can live a healthy life with just one kidney, sustaining life needs some kidney function.

The kidneys have an essential role in heart failure, especially in maintaining **fluid balance** throughout the circulatory system. They also have a function in **blood pressure** and maintaining **salt and mineral levels** within the body.

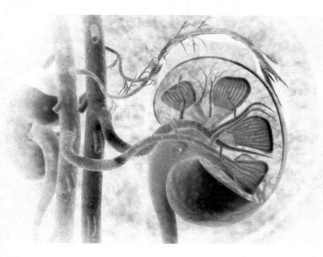

The kidneys are important in maintaining fluid balance, blood pressure and salt and mineral levels within the body.

The body's **renal system** is essentially a filtration system. To begin to understand it, let's think of it as a pool filtration system as represented by the following diagram:

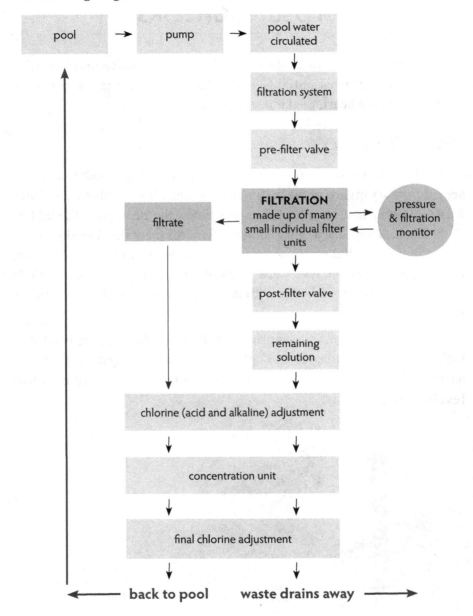

filtration system: swimming pool

Now, replace the pool system with the body's renal system:

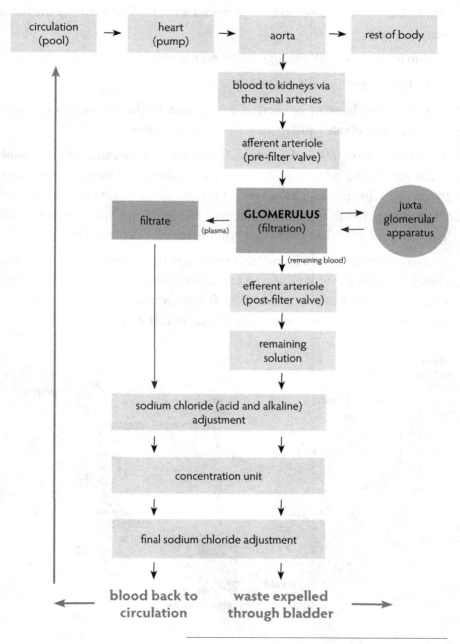

filtration system: body's renal system

Each kidney is made up of about one million filtering units called **nephrons**. Each nephron includes a **glomerulus** – a cluster of tiny blood capillaries (the filter) – and a **tubule**. A blood vessel runs alongside the tubule. Larger molecules (such as proteins) and blood cells, stay in the blood vessel.

The nephrons work through a two-step process:

- the glomerulus filters the blood and
- the tubule returns needed substances to the blood and removes wastes. Wastes and extra water become urine.

As blood flows into each nephron it enters the glomerulus. The thin walls of the glomerulus allow smaller molecules, wastes, and fluid, mostly water, to pass into the tubule. The tubule returns needed substances – most of the water, along with minerals and nutrients needed by the body – to the blood. The remaining fluid and wastes left in the tubule become urine.

Blood flows into each kidney through the **renal artery.** This large blood vessel branches into smaller and smaller blood vessels until the blood reaches the nephrons. After filtration, it flows into increasingly larger veins until it flows out of the kidney through the **renal vein.**

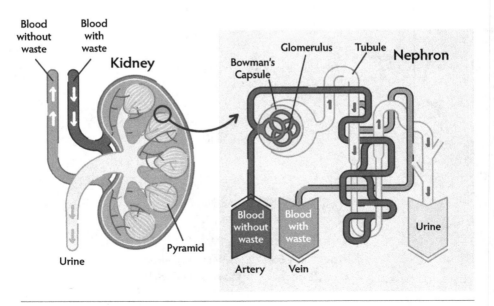

nephron anatomy

Blood circulates through the body's kidneys many times a day – 4.5 liters per minute. Most of the water and other substances that filter through the glomeruli are returned to the blood by the tubules. Only a relatively small amount becomes urine.

The kidneys feature prominently throughout this book.

the lungs

A close link exists between the heart and the lungs. These two organs are interdependent and connected physically through the circulatory system. The lungs and their associated respiratory system provide the life-giving oxygen from the air to the blood, which, pumped by the heart, nourishes the body. The lungs then expel the waste product, carbon dioxide, from the body. These two sponge-like organs are located on either side of the chest (the thorax) and are close to the heart.

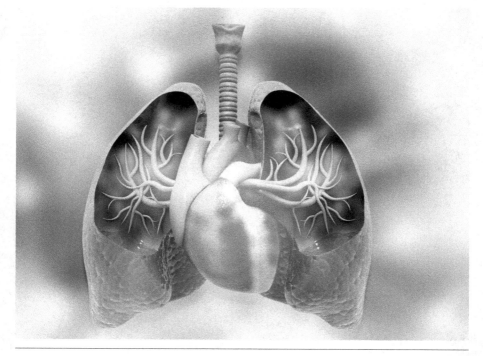

the lungs in relation to the heart

Cardiac failure involves the interaction of

- the **heart** (that pumps the life-giving oxygen around the body)
- the **kidneys** (that help maintain the body's fluid balance, blood pressure, salt and mineral levels) and
- the **lungs** and their associated **respiratory system** (that provide the body with oxygen and remove carbon dioxide).

The heart, the kidneys and the lungs are connected by the circulatory system.

---

[3]   *Kidney Health Australia (https://kidney.org.au/your-kidneys/prevent/what-your-kidneys-do)*

TERRY'S JOURNEY

"She'll be right mate!" but it wasn't!!!

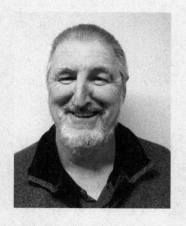

I am a 62-year-old male with more than 45 years' experience working in the mental health/disability industry as a registered nurse, both hands-on and as a manager. My heart problems were a double whammy. Historically, as a nurse, we make the worst kind of patient and, as a male I have the "she'll be right, mate", "all's good, nothing to worry about", "it'll go away tomorrow" attitude. Well, surprise, surprise! It wasn't alright, and it didn't go away, not until I received expert care from my family GP of 40 years, my learned cardiologist and his cardiac care team.

As a young person, you worry about getting good school results, finding a suitable and rewarding career, raising a family the best way you can with your partner and all the time planning for your retirement. Then, when the time comes, you are faced with another significant quandary. What is the best way to retire for the benefit of your family and yourself? I was in the process of planning my transition to retirement. The intention was to move from full-time work to part-time hours, to then working as a casual nurse.

I first noticed that I was having small heart palpitations while at work but thought nothing of it. I put it down to feeling a little stressed and overwhelmed about planning the next phase of my life. Then, one day at work, I noticed that my glasses in my shirt pocket were moving and I could feel my heart beating rapidly in my chest. Naturally, I felt my pulse which showed an irregular rhythm around 150 to 170 beats per minute. "S—t," I thought, "that's a bit high. Just take a few deep breaths and relax." I didn't feel any other symptoms such as dizziness, spots before my eyes, pain or discomfort in the chest; there was no raised jugular vein or clammy skin.

Then the treating doctors arrived on my unit for medical rounds, so my mind was diverted to other matters, and I soon forgot about it.

While this episode came and went, I had noticed over several weeks and was told by my 'better half', that I was lagging when we were walking our dog. Yes, I felt a little breathless when exerting myself too quickly but again thought, "All's good; I'm just a little unfit". Then, on one walk, I had to physically stop on several occasions to catch my breath, especially while going up a small incline. This breathlessness had both of us a little concerned. I made an appointment with my GP, who performed an ECG in his rooms.

His diagnosis was that I was carrying excessive fluid around the heart, suffering atrial fibrillation (AF) and was in the early stages of congestive cardiac failure (CCF). I had thought that I was asymptomatic of any significant health issue. He promptly contacted a cardiac specialist at my local hospital who graciously agreed to see me that afternoon. The cardiologist ordered a series of blood tests, an echocardiogram, a cardiac CT, and commenced me on several heart medications to alleviate the symptoms. I was also admitted, as a day patient, on two occasions, to undergo a cardioversion procedure for the AF. This was to bring my heartbeat back into a normal rhythm and rate. Thankfully, it has done so for the past two years.

Now, it's all water under the bridge and life is almost back to normal. With my regular annual heart check-up and medication review with my cardiologist and his team and the ongoing support of my wife, I hope to remain in reasonably good health. ♥

Three significant systems within the body link the heart, the kidneys and the lungs. We need to know something about them.

chapter 4
CHALLENGING THE BODY'S FLUID BALANCE

At any suggestion of a threat to its fluid balance or blood volume, the body reacts. One pathway is through the autonomic nervous system (ANS) and the other is via chemical-based channel systems.

Specialized pressure receptors located within the large blood vessels in the chest and neck react to any changes in the body's **fluid volume** and **pressure**. They feed back this change to the lower part of the brain which then influences the **autonomic nervous system**.

Depending on whether the receptors recognize an increase or decrease in blood volume and pressure within the body, the ANS then regulates blood vessel relaxation or constriction and nervous stimulation to the kidneys and the heart. This ANS response is entirely automatic, meaning that the body responds in a way that we are unaware of and over which we have no direct cognitive control.

The two **chemical-based channel systems** act mainly through the **kidneys**.

Body fluid balance is primarily a function of the kidneys and, in particular, is regulated by the **juxtaglomerular apparatus** (*juxta,* near; *glomerulus,* the filtration unit; *apparatus,* a collection of specialized cells). This chemical-based system influences the heart. The juxtaglomerular apparatus responds to local blood pressure and to the ANS input, the latter reflecting the specialized pressure receptors of the large blood vessels. The juxtaglomerular cells increase fluid volume and pressure by acting on a chemical messenger system in the body called the **renin-angiotensin-aldosterone system** (RAAS) so that the body **retains** fluid. This fluid retention in the body keeps sodium and water in the kidneys and stimulates the sympathetic nervous system (SNS) to **increase** blood pressure through increased vascular tone (by constricting the arteries).

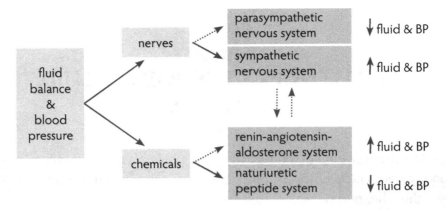

The other chemical-based system takes pressure off the **heart**; it is the **natriuretic peptide system** (NPS) (*naturesis*, fluid leaves the body by increased urination; *peptide*, a mini protein). This system induces **naturesis** that causes the kidneys to **release** sodium and water, which **lowers** the blood pressure and so **reduces** pressure on the heart.

Let's look at each of these systems in more detail.

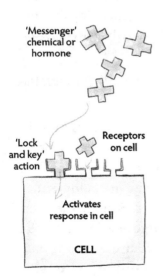

RECEPTORS

Receptors are the way that hormones or chemical messengers in the bloodstream interact with their target cells. **A receptor is simply a docking station that is specific to the hormone or chemical in question.**

A lock/key relationship exists between a receptor and its designated chemical messenger. Once the chemical messenger sits on its specific docking station located on the cell surface, the docking station initiates a series of further chemical reactions within the cell to activate the effect of the hormone or chemical messenger.

For those of us old enough to remember the coin-operated lolly dispensers, think of 1) the coin as the messenger, 2) the slot as the receptor, and 3) the turning knob that releases a lolly as the action, remembering that it has to be the right coin for the right slot.

the autonomic nervous system

We can be aware of wanting to undertake a very deliberate movement: moving a hand, moving two hands, snapping a finger, looking to the left, looking to the right. Such **intentional** actions are generated within the **parietal lobe** of the **cerebral cortex**, also known as the **cerebrum**. The parietal lobe sits below the skull and just behind the temples. The nerves in the parietal lobe connect with the muscles that we want to action. Very deliberate. Very conscious.

Then, there is the nerve function that occurs without us giving the action a thought: blood pressure changing, heart rate varying, our gut digesting a meal. For the most part, we are **not conscious** of these actions and yet they are critical for our body's function. This is the **autonomic nervous system** (ANS). It is automatic; we don't need to think about it.

The ANS has two main parts: one looks after actions that speed us up and one looks after actions which slow us down. Continuing our car analogy, it is somewhat like the accelerator and brake. The 'accelerator' is the **sympathetic nervous system** (SNS) which prepares our body for 'fight and flight' and kicks in when the body is challenged in any way. The 'brake' is the **parasympathetic nervous system** (PNS) that helps us slow down, to 'digest and relax'.

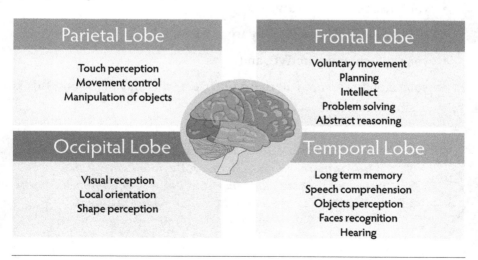

Parietal Lobe

Touch perception
Movement control
Manipulation of objects

Frontal Lobe

Voluntary movement
Planning
Intellect
Problem solving
Abstract reasoning

Occipital Lobe

Visual reception
Local orientation
Shape perception

Temporal Lobe

Long term memory
Speech comprehension
Objects perception
Faces recognition
Hearing

The cerebral cortex is the largest part of the human brain and consists of the frontal lobe, the parietal lobe, the occipital lobe and the temporal lobe and is associated with higher brain functions such as thought and action.

If you are under attack, the **SNS** comes into play:

- **your eyes will dilate** so that you can see everything, even in the dark;

- **your saliva glands will stop working**, because you are not going to be eating;

- more **blood flows to the lungs** so you can breathe better;

- **your heart rate increases**, so, as the heart beats with greater strength, your blood pressure rises;

- **blood flow to the gut slows** and **digestion shuts down** so your energy reserves are directed to the 'fight or flight' response;

- **blood flow to the muscles increases**, giving you more strength, and

- your **kidneys** will act to preserve fluid and maintain blood pressure.

The **PNS** does the opposite:

- your eyes will **constrict**;

- you will **salivate**;

- your heart rate will **slow**;

- blood will be **diverted away** from the muscles;

- your gut will **keep active,** and

- your blood pressure will **drop** (if severe, you may black-out; this is a 'simple faint').

The PNS works quite hard in the middle of the night. While you are in deep sleep, your heart rate slows and your gut digests whatever you have eaten before going to bed. This is central to having a regular bowel.

homeostasis for fluid balance

A significant **automatic** response within the body is **fluid balance**. We don't need to think about it. We feel thirsty and we drink a glass of water, then we go to the toilet and pass urine. We don't need to measure what fluid is taken in and what fluid goes out as the body is very clever at regulating that for us. Several systems come together to ensure that the body's fluid remains in constant balance.

One of the key elements here is the involvement of pressure receptors or **baroreceptors.** These receptors measure the **barometric pressure**, which is the pressure within the fluid of the vasculature of the body's large blood vessels. The baroreceptors are found in two locations.

Our first location of interest is in the **aortic arch**. This is situated just past the heart's aortic valve, where the blood starts to flow from the heart to the rest of the body. The other is in the **carotid arteries.** These arteries are located on each side of the neck and supply blood to the head and the brain. Baroreceptors are positioned on the carotid arteries at the bulb, also called the carotid sinus. This is where the carotid arteries divide into two branches. One branch supplies blood to the brain and the other branch runs on the outside of the skull to supply blood to the head (face, neck and scalp).

In both positions, the baroreceptors are constantly testing the blood pressure going to significant organs – the heart, the brain and the kidneys – and sending feedback to the medulla, the lower part of the brain that links with the ANS acting on the arteries and the kidneys.

As an example, if the baroreceptors near the heart feel the blood pressure is decreasing, a signal goes to the medulla. If the medulla 'thinks' the person has lost fluid or the blood pressure is too low, it sends signals through the SNS to tighten up the arteries, which message the kidneys to improve filtration. This feedback loop continually tests and evaluates in order to maintain an ideal fluid balance within the body.

Also, as part of fluid balance, the body needs to maintain a constant concentration of different **salts**. Our interest is sodium or sodium chloride, commonly known as table salt. The body needs to keep its 'saltiness' stable. If there is too much salt, the body becomes 'pickled'. **Not good**. Too little salt and the body's tissues swell up, like your fingertips if you spend too long in the bath. **Not good.** So, there is an ideal concentration of sodium that the body keeps very carefully regulated. Sensors in the brain tell us if the salt levels rise too much. We are thirsty. Water 'in'. The kidneys regulate both sodium **loss**, which takes water with it (water 'out'), and sodium **reabsorption**, which keeps water 'in'.

These continuously-occurring processes are looking after vital, life-determining functions such as blood pressure, heart rate, heart-pumping functions, digestion and kidney filtration. The maintenance of these pre-set determinants is called **homeostasis** (*homeo*, similar; *stasis*, being stable; *homeostasis*, the capacity of the body to maintain stability of diverse internal variables).

The ANS, responding to baroreceptor feedback, influences body responses that keep us in balance, to maintain the body's homeostasis.

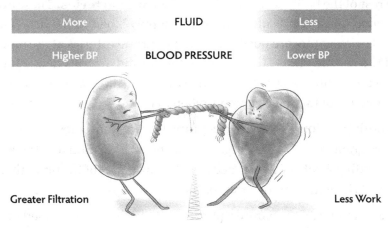

kidney – heart tensions

chemical messenger systems

The above description of the ANS is a **neural** or nerve-based response to a challenge to the fluid balance in the body. As discussed earlier, the other response involves the two main chemical messenger systems within the body: the **renin-angiotensin-aldosterone system** (RAAS), which regulates blood pressure through the kidneys, and the **natriuretic peptide system** (NPS), which takes pressure off the heart.

These two systems produce chemical messengers that flow through the body, helping to control how the body responds to any fluid disturbance, whether it be too little or too much fluid. The messengers also help the body's response to any threat to the **kidneys** not receiving the blood flow they require to maintain **adequate filtration**. These chemical systems work together to maintain the balance of fluid and blood pressure within the body to ensure that the kidneys and heart function optimally.

Step 1 – Filtration

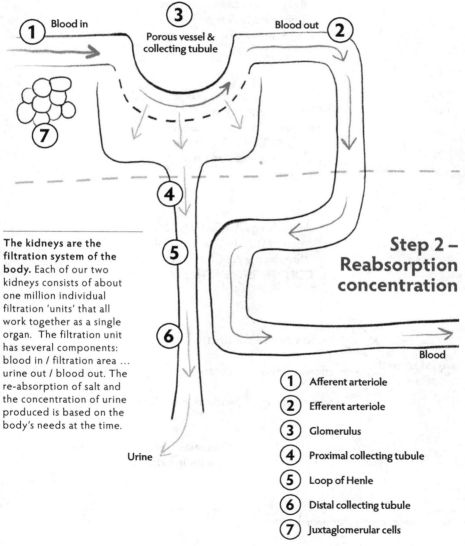

The kidneys are the filtration system of the body. Each of our two kidneys consists of about one million individual filtration 'units' that all work together as a single organ. The filtration unit has several components: blood in / filtration area ... urine out / blood out. The re-absorption of salt and the concentration of urine produced is based on the body's needs at the time.

Blood in

3 Porous vessel & collecting tubule

Blood out

Step 2 – Reabsorption concentration

Blood

Urine

1 Afferent arteriole

2 Efferent arteriole

3 Glomerulus

4 Proximal collecting tubule

5 Loop of Henle

6 Distal collecting tubule

7 Juxtaglomerular cells

63

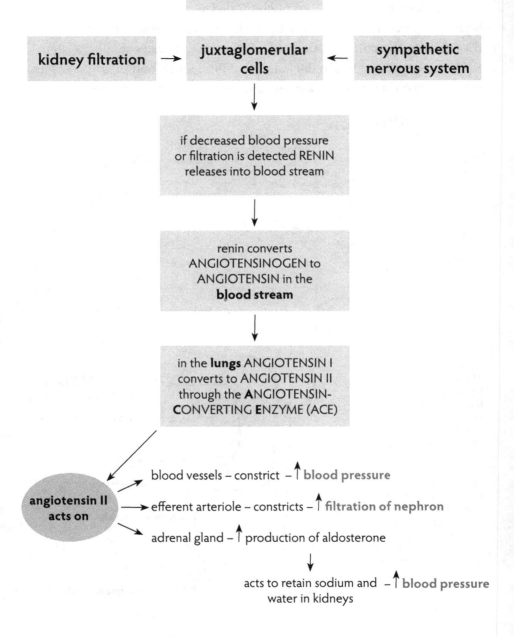

the renin-angiotensin-aldosterone system

The renin-angiotensin-aldosterone system (RAAS) principally looks after the **kidneys.**

Specialized cells within the kidney, the **juxtaglomerular cells,** continually monitor the kidneys' blood pressure, checking that the kidneys have enough blood flow to filter off sufficient fluid to produce urine. Located very near the collecting tubules where the filtration occurs, these cells are sensitive to changes in blood flow or pressure. When the blood flow decreases, they become active and release the chemical, **renin.** Renin causes a series of other chemical interactions to occur (which will be discussed in more detail later) that stimulate the kidneys to restore filtration and blood pressure and return the body to homeostasis. One activator is the SNS, triggered by the baroreceptors. Another could be that the person has lost blood and so the juxtaglomerular cells receive a message to maintain blood pressure required by the kidneys for continuous filtration.

When the cells release renin, the chemical cuts, or cleaves a protein, called **angiotensinogen**, that is already present in the bloodstream, having been produced by the liver.

I was hoping you wouldn't ask why the liver produces it. My take is that the liver is a busy manufacturing organ; an organ where a lot of synthesis and production happens. So, I guess if you're going to make something in a factory, the liver is as good a factory as any in which to make proteins.

Renin modifies angiotensinogen into **angiotensin I (AT1)** which is now floating around the body in the bloodstream. As it moves through the lungs, within the lining of the lungs, there is another enzyme, or protein, that cleaves angiotensin I into **angiotensin II (AT2)**. This protein is called **angiotensin-converting enzyme (ACE).**

(AT2) now floats around the body and can act on two sets of receptors, the angiotensin I (AT1) receptors and the angiotensin II (AT2) receptors. These receptors are located in various organs in the body. The AT2 receptor, which is found in the heart, blood vessels, kidneys, adrenal cortex, lungs, circumventricular organs of brain, basal ganglia, and brainstem, mediates the vasoconstrictor effects. Of most interest here are the **AT2 receptors** as they act to keep blood pressure up and maintain kidney function. These receptors lead to **vasoconstriction** within certain arteries of the body. This **raises** the pressure within the whole circulatory system and, so, **increases filtration pressure** within the kidneys to keep them working in peak condition.

AT2 acts on the **efferent arteriole** that is on the exit side, or the far side, of the glomerular filtration system. If this artery **constricts**, the pressure within the glomerulus **increases**, boosting the filtration. *(refer to 'post filter valve' in the filtration system diagrams in chapter 3, pages 50 and 51)*

This is important as angiotensin-converting enzyme inhibitor (or ACE inhibitor) drugs play a significant role in treating cardiac failure.

AT2 also directly increases the amount of **aldosterone**, a hormone that acts on the kidney to alter sodium (salt) re-absorption. AT2 works at the adrenal gland to increase aldosterone release. As the body cannot hold sodium alone – it would become far too salty – the body needs to hold water with it, which, in turn, increases the blood volume in the body.

The role of AT2 in the renin-angiotensin-aldosterone system is to protect kidney function by increasing blood pressure through the body via vasoconstriction and fluid retention. It increases kidney filtration by constricting the efferent arteriole that leaves the filtration unit, and it increases the amount of sodium reabsorbed into the body, ensuring more water is kept in the body so that the body maintains fluid and pressure.

Constriction of the efferent arteriole reduces the blood's ability to leave the glomerulus system, the blood backs up, the pressure increases and, so, the filtration increases.

the natriuretic peptide system

The natriuretic peptide system (NPS) principally **supports cardiac function**, helping the heart to work with reduced strain.

In this system, particular **peptides** (mini hormones, small strings of the body's basic building blocks, amino acids, held together by peptide bonds) are released from the heart when the heart is under strain. **Natriuretic** refers to passing urine or fluid loss. So, this natriuretic peptide system produces peptides that cause a natriuresis if the heart is under stress.

When triggered, natriuretic peptides perform some significant functions that support and protect the heart. They:

- **cause natriuresis**, fluid loss, which makes the person pass more urine, taking pressure off the heart.

- **reduce blood pressure**, due to vasodilation, or widening of the blood vessels, which takes pressure off the heart. The more vasoconstriction (narrowing) of the arteries, the higher the resistance against which the heart pumps. So, when natriuretic peptides widen the arteries, they help relieve undue pressure on the heart.

- **decrease sympathetic tone,** or the autonomic component, of the nervous system which drives the 'fight or flight' response that is known to put a strain on the heart.

- **decrease aldosterone**, one of the hormones which makes the kidneys retain sodium. If the kidneys retain sodium, they retain fluid (water), and that increases blood volume, which increases pressures within the system. By diminishing the effect of aldosterone, sodium is lost, fluid is lost, and less strain is put on the heart.

- **have a role in reducing inflammation** and fibrosis within the heart. In the long term, natriuretic peptides protect the integrity of the heart muscle, reducing the likelihood of damage through inflammation and subsequent fibrosis, or scarring.

- **alter the way the heart responds to strain**, reducing the remodeling, which can be detrimental when the heart is under load. If the heart is under strain for any length of time, pumping too hard against blood pressure or even pumping too hard against a valve, the heart responds by changing structurally (morphologically). The muscle thickens (like a body builder's muscles morphologically change; they get bigger). Natriuretic peptides diminish that response. Keeping the heart in its normal shape is very beneficial for the patient.

The renin-angiotensin-aldosterone system and the natriuretic peptide system are like the 'yin and yang' of a body in cardiac and renal balance, and when they become misaligned in cardiac failure, they are very good targets for therapies that can adjust the way these systems work.

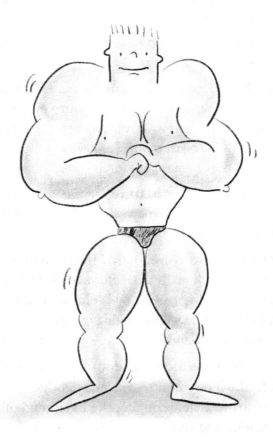

If the heart is under strain for any length of time, the heart responds by changing structurally (morphologically). Like a body builder's muscles morphologically change, the heart muscle can change. Natriuretic peptides diminish that response.

the autonomic nervous system

- regulates fluid volume based on feedback from baroreceptors in the chest and neck
- does not have direct cognitive influence
- consists of

the sympathetic nervous system (fight or flight – 'accelerator')	the parasympathetic nervous system (rest or digest – 'brake')
eyes dilate	eyes constrict
saliva glands stop working	salivation
more blood flows to the lungs and muscles	blood diverted from muscles
heart rate increases, BP rises	heart rate slows, BP drops
blood flow to gut slows; digestion shuts down	gut keeps active
kidney function changes	

fluid balance

- baroreceptors measure the pressure of the fluid within the large blood vessels, the aorta and the carotid arteries
- homeostasis automatically checks that the body's fluid is in balance
- the body's 'saltiness' needs to be stable

(continued next page)

two chemical messenger systems

- renin-angiotensin-aldosterone-system (RAAS)
  - **looks after the kidneys**
  - juxtaglomerular cells (in the kidneys) release renin when there is a loss of blood
  - renin cleaves angiotensinogen (already in the bloodstream) into angiotensin I which cleaves into angiotensin II, by a protein called angiotensin-converting enzyme (ACE)
- **natriuretic peptide system (NPS)**
  - **looks after the heart**
  - particular peptides are released from the heart when the heart is under strain. They
    - cause natriuresis
    - reduce blood pressure
    - decrease sympathetic tone
    - decrease aldosterone
    - have a decisive role in reducing inflammation and fibrosis
    - alter the way the heart responds to strain

Now that we know about the systems and the relationships involved, what is cardiac failure?

THE HEART

WHEN IT FAILS

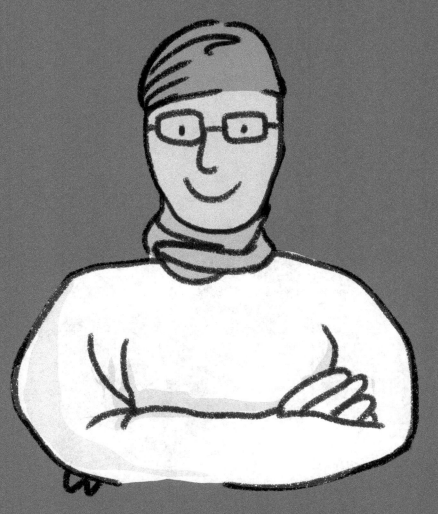

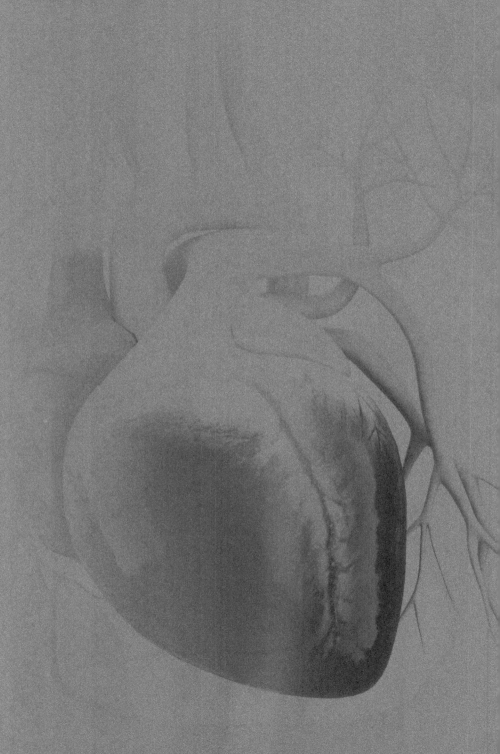

EMMA'S JOURNEY

a renewed life

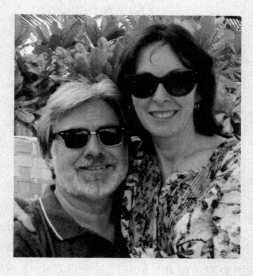

Hi, my name is Emma; it is 2019, and I am 60 years old. I write this in the hope my story may help anyone who is suffering from heart failure and is fearful of the pathway ahead.

In 2014, I underwent two lumpectomies that resulted in a diagnosis of breast cancer stage 3 grade 3, with two tumors found in my right breast and three tumors in my lymph glands. Six months of horrific chemotherapy followed, and then, immediately, six weeks of radiotherapy. At the time, my elderly mother was living with us – my husband, Peter, and I – and needed care. In the midst of all of this, the world as I had known it, stopped. What would be the 'new normal', and how would we make sense of it?

We just 'got on with it', with the lion's share of caring falling on Peter's shoulders. He did this with such grace and so willingly that he sacrificed his PhD studies to look after us both. When my treatment finished, my heart looked stable and appeared to be normal. Although I was told to be careful as the chemotherapy used for cancer treatment can cause damage to the heart, I thought I might be fortunate and dodge this bullet.

I returned to music teaching in a junior school in 2016. Teaching the joys of music to young children was my passion. It was great to be alive, and every day was a new gift. I felt reasonably strong although I often felt tired, possibly an after-effect of the chemo as well as a side-effect of the hormone suppressant medication, arimidex, I was taking every day. As my mother's condition progressed slowly, Peter relaxed a little now that I was back at work. My general health was okay and I was looking forward to the 11 music concerts for the end-of-year celebrations. This number of concerts was not a remarkable load in the life of a music teacher, and I had done it many times in my 30-plus years of teaching. What happened next would genuinely test my faith. People, circumstances and an amazing medical team became my angels in an act of Divine intervention. My time was not up yet!

In November 2016, I visited my GP to discuss a very consistent, niggly cough that I had developed. I could only speak a few words at a time before breaking into a coughing spasm. Walking any distance or on an incline, including climbing stairs, had become challenging. I thought it was end-of-year job fatigue and, after all, it was not that long since my recovery from breast cancer. While I dismissed these symptoms and soldiered on, the ridiculous dry cough would not go away.

One morning, a colleague pulled me aside to say how she thought I was looking very pale and that my cough sounded like her grandmother's cough. What was significant here was that her grandmother's cough was a result of her having heart failure after she had had breast cancer. My cough sounded the same. I promised to visit my GP.

The GP was curious; I had been doing so well in my recovery. The symptoms I described were:

- persistent, niggly coughing when speaking or moving about;
- feeling tired, often;
- playing the piano was like lifting lead weights on my arms;
- I could only climb three stairs at a time before pausing with coughing and fatigue;
- I could hardly muster a singing voice, and
- while moving about, I was getting short of breath and sweating more than usual.

And I continued to cough, cough, cough.

The GP ordered an electrocardiogram (ECG) with the results read immediately in the surgery. Although there were some issues, they were *not enough to put me in hospital. "Go home and rest" was the advice given. That night, however, my GP phoned me at home and recommended that I visit a heart specialist. She had already arranged a consultation for the next day. So off we went, not aware of what was happening. An echocardiogram (echo) and another ECG were done on arrival at the specialist's rooms. The echo technician was so compassionate and caring while performing the procedure. She, of course, could not tell me what she had found, but I knew I was in trouble. What was going on?*

My husband and I then met the heart specialist, and he revealed with certainty that I was in a state of severe heart failure, probably due to the chemotherapy that I had received. I did not hear much after that as the shock was significant. The specialist quickly picked up on my panicked state. As he started to go through what options I had, he explained that he would endeavor to treat the heart failure with drug therapy. The effect of the drugs would not be immediate, he said, but could work in the longer term. I quickly focused on what was necessary to improve.

This very kind specialist taught me how to monitor my heart. I needed to keep a daily journal of medications, to take regular blood pressure readings, weigh myself morning and night and record these findings. Drug names needed to be learned and, of course, the drugs taken: micardis, bisoprolol, spironolactone and furosemide. Already feeling completely exhausted, this took some discipline. Throughout my breast cancer treatment, my mantra had been, it's not what happens to you in life, it's how you handle it. *This kicked in again, and Peter stepped in to assist in every way he could. For this, I remain grateful.*

I still had two end-of-year concerts to complete, and diligently prepared. Feeling worse than usual, I went back to the heart specialist and was hospitalized immediately. My blood work indicated some difficulties of which I was oblivious. Peter brought my concert clothing to the hospital so that I could complete the afternoon concert and then the evening concert. How that happened is anybody's guess. I could barely stand in my high-heeled shoes. As soon as the concert was over, I was back in the hospital, placed on a drip, and more blood work undertaken. I was unaware of how sick I was. While in the hospital for several days, my tablet dosages were readjusted. Slowly, I regained some strength.

Christmas came and went without incident as my mother and husband lovingly supported me. Three weeks passed. The various readings were recorded in the journal, but I was still very lethargic. As the new school year was about to start, I revisited the heart specialist. Another echo revealed significant fluid build-up between the heart and the walls of my left lung. The fluid had to be drained. In the hospital, on Friday before the new school term started, 1.4 liters of fluid were drained from my chest cavity that is between the heart and the lung.

To say that I felt great after this was an understatement. I haven't looked back!

Resuming my music teaching with gusto began the new journey of living, albeit with breast cancer hormone therapy, lymphedema and heart failure! Yes, it is achievable when all the checks and balances are followed.

I am so grateful for the wonderful support given to me by my husband and my mum over these years as they, too, embraced the 'new normal'. My GP and the heart specialist have given us tremendous support, as such a journey is faced by the family, not only the patient. The medicos have been there whenever I needed them. Not only did they save my life, but they have also given me the tools I need to live my renewed life.

It is now the end of 2019. I am happily retired. I spent this past year caring for my mother before she died, with Peter there every step of the way. I am so grateful to be alive and to be able to enjoy each new day. My heart is stable, and I continue to take my heart medications and hormone therapy.

If anyone needs living proof that there is life after cancer and heart failure, it's me. My prayers were answered as the angels helped me at every turn. This journey is a testament to faith and the considered and wise choices that were made by my medical team. It's because of both that I am here today. Remember, it's not what happens to you that defines you as a human being; it's how you deal with it. ♥

Congestive cardiac failure (CCF) is the term that refers to the retention of the fluid that occurs in heart failure. It leads to fluid overload of the body, creating 'congestion'. CCF requires timely medical attention as the heart has lost its ability to pump properly, causing a flow-on of effects. Depriving itself, other body organs and tissues of oxygen and nutrients, extra fluid builds up in various parts of the body causing swelling, and including the lungs where it causes shortness of breath.

types of heart failure

There are several types of heart failure:

- **left-sided, or left ventricular (LV) heart failure**, in which the left-hand side of the heart has impaired function

  - **HF with Reduced Ejection Fraction** (HFrEF), also called **systolic** failure, in which the left ventricle **does not contract properly** and, so, cannot pump enough blood into the circulation, and

  - **HF with Preserved Ejection Fraction** (HFpEF), also called **diastolic** failure or diastolic dysfunction, in which the left ventricle **loses its ability to relax.** When the muscle becomes stiff, the heart cannot fill with blood correctly during the rest phase between each beat, and

- **right-sided heart failure,** which is most commonly a result of left-side failure. When the fluid pressure backs up through the lungs, it causes the right side of the heart to compensate then eventually decompensate.

classifications

There are three main classification distinctions used concerning heart failure:

- **time**
- **function**
- **degree of incapacity brought on by breathlessness**.

The **time** relates to whether the heart failure has developed quickly (acute) or slowly (chronic). The **function** classification is based on the ejection fraction (reduced, preserved or moderate). The New York Heart Association Classification of Cardiac Failure[4] guides the understanding of **incapacity.**

living with heart failure

Although the heart function of some individuals may recover after an initial insult, there is no specific cure. However, the damage may be mitigated, and the deterioration stabilized so that the patient can continue to lead a fulfilling life.

The prevalence of heart failure is increasing, due, at least in part, to the **ageing population**, as well as **better survival rates** in patients with cardiovascular disease.

Treatment includes a range of drug therapies, cardiac implants (devices), surgical procedures, and, in extreme cases, heart transplantation. Most of the treatments involve multidisciplinary management in which experts combine their knowledge and skills for the patient's best outcome.

[4]   *Adapted from Dolgin M, Association NYH, Fox AC, Gorlin R, Levin RI, New York Heart Association. Criteria Committee. Nomenclature and criteria for diagnosis of diseases of the heart and great vessels. 9th ed. Boston, MA: Lippincott Williams and Wilkins; March 1, 1994. Original source: Criteria Committee, New York Heart Association, Inc. Diseases of the Heart and Blood Vessels. Nomenclature and Criteria for diagnosis, 6th edition Boston, Little, Brown and Co. 1964, p 114.*

chapter 5
SHORT OF BREATH? PUFFY ANKLES?

From an historical perspective, cardiac failure has been recognized for thousands of years. Individuals having the symptoms of cardiac failure – swelling in the extremities, particularly the legs, and shortness of breath, – was recorded by the Babylonians, the Egyptians and the Greeks. So, the medical profession has been observing the process of people retaining fluid and suffering the consequences for a long time. However, it wasn't until the end of the 17th century that the combined symptoms of retaining fluid and the associated shortness of breath were named 'dropsy'.

Although the features were observed more frequently and became more widely recognized in the 18th century, it took until end of the 19th century for English physicians, John Blackall (1771-1860) and Richard Bright (1789-1858), to advance the understanding of the process of fluid retention. They recognized there were two sets of circumstances that could lead to the situation. The first set involved heart problems and the second set involved kidney problems. Both lead to an imbalance of fluid within the body. They also recognized that salt and water were central to this process.

Efforts then focused on trying to control the condition by removing the fluid and thus helping the symptoms. Two main ways to do this evolved. One was by altering secretions or making people release more fluid, either through diaphoresis, which made them sweat, or through the loss of fluid through their bowels, using purgatives. The other way the body removed the fluid was by direct means: some patients would undergo a process of bleeding where blood was taken from the veins; some underwent leeching, and some, lancing. These were the practices for many years. It wasn't until the post-World War I era that doctors started to look towards agents that used mercury as a base active ingredient as potential diuretics. These original agents, although they had some efficacy, were not successful. The development of currently-used diuretic agents did not occur until the end of the 1940s and into the 1950s.

Modern diuretics are agents that keep salt in the urine. This liberation of salt and water from the body allows the kidneys and the urine to be the source of the release of the extra fluid which collects as part of cardiac failure or from deranged renal function. Our focus will be the cardiac failure component, as renal failure leading to swelling is a very different matter.

....

A BRIEF HISTORY OF UNDERSTANDING HEART FAILURE

1628   *William Harvey describes the circulation*

end of 17th century

the term, 'dropsy', is coined for people with symptoms of fluid retention and shortness of breath

1785   *William Withering publishes an account of medical use of digitalis*

around the turn of the century

John Blackall and Richard Bright advance the understanding of fluid retention

1819   *René Laennec invents the stethoscope*

1895   *Wilhelm Röntgen discovers x-rays*

1920   *organomercurial diuretics are first used*

1954   *Inge Edler and Hellmuth Hertz use ultrasound to image cardiac structures*

1958   *thiazide diuretics are introduced*

1967   *Christiaan Barnard performs first human heart transplant*

1987   *CONSENSUS-I study shows unequivocal survival benefit of angiotensin-converting enzyme inhibitors in severe heart failure*

1995   *European Society of Cardiology publishes guidelines for diagnosing heart failure*

....

symptoms

Patients who have features of cardiac failure tend to describe **shortness of breath mainly on exertion**. Often, they notice climbing hills or climbing stairs or carrying their groceries as the activity that triggers their awareness that they are more breathless than usual. They may describe **fatigue** or lethargy or lack of motivation to undertake activities because of their shortness of breath. These patients are also likely to report some **swelling**, particularly in their legs, and, if their condition is more serious, in their tummies. Sometimes, as in Emma's experience, they may present with a persistent **cough.**

Two particular circumstances seen with cardiac failure-induced shortness of breath are **position-related.**

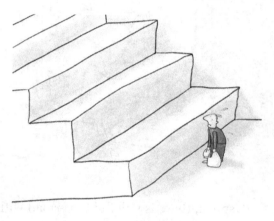

So commonly, when patients are sitting or standing **upright**, the fluid within the body tends to be drawn, by gravity, to the lower extremities, their legs. When in a sitting or standing position, the lungs, relative to the fluid balance that is in the body, remain relatively free of the extra fluid that has accumulated.

It sounds a bit odd, but it is useful to think of excess fluid slushing around the body under the influence of gravity.

In contrast, when a person lies down **flat**, or almost flat, in a recumbent position, and he or she becomes short of breath, this is **orthopnea** (*ortho*, upright; *pnea,* breathing).

The circulation's excess fluid being held in the lower extremities by gravity moves to the chest and causes congestion within the lungs. Sitting upright improves the situation almost immediately.

Another related condition is **paroxysmal nocturnal dyspnea** (PND), a precursor to orthopnea. PND is shortness of breath that comes

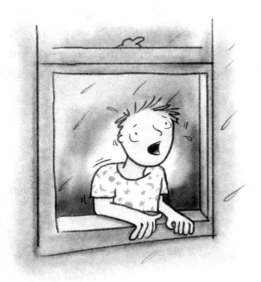

somewhat unexpectedly in the middle of the night. Patients describe going to bed without any problems. They have several hours of comfortable sleep. Then, suddenly, sleep is interrupted, and they wake with shortness of breath. A feeling of suffocation provokes anxiety and fear. These patients sit up, get out of bed and often open a window — fresh air and standing help to relieve their symptoms.

With paroxysmal nocturnal dyspnea, there is still fluid overload within the body, but not to the same extent as orthopnea, and some of that overload is held within the tissues, not just within the circulation. When the person lies down to rest overnight, the fluid moves from the tissues into the circulation. As the circulatory volume increases, it flows back to the chest where it causes congestion and the shortness of breath, and wakes up the person. Altering the posture starts to shift the fluid away from the lungs, and that brings relief to the breathing. Patients report that they find relief by standing up, going to a window and breathing in fresh air.

Please consult your GP or your primary care provider if you have any of the above symptoms.

To bring standardization to discussions about cardiac failure, the **New York Heart Association (NYHA) Classification of Cardiac Failure** categorizes the breathing symptoms of a patient. These stages are discussed more fully in a subsequent chapter.

IMPORTANT POINTS

- Cardiac failure has been observed and documented for thousands of years.

- Understanding and treatment have evolved beyond leeches and laxatives.

- Modern diuretic agents take salt and water from the body through the kidneys to help balance congestion within the circulation.

- Cardiac failure can include positional issues, including lying down, and the patient waking from sleep.

- The New York Heart Association Classification of Cardiac Failure provides a reference for discussion among medical practitioners.

So, what causes cardiac failure?

chapter 6
CAUSES OF CARDIAC FAILURE

Cardiac failure (CF) occurs when the pumping capacity of the heart does not match the cardiac output required by the body.

The heart can fail in several ways:

1. **integrity of the muscle**. Coronary artery disease causes lack of blood flow to the heart. Toxins, infection and inflammation affect the heart. Unwanted substances can infiltrate the heart and stop the muscle from working correctly, while metabolic and genetic issues can also come into play.

2. **abnormal load.** Blood pressure, problems with the valves, and congenital issues need to be considered, as do too much fluid in the system and if the body has an altered need for a dynamic circulatory system (a high output state), and

3. **abnormal timing**. If the electrical system of the heart is out of synchronization, the heart rate can be too fast or too slow, and this affects the pumping capacity of the heart.

integrity of the muscle

Coronary artery disease, or ischemic heart disease, is one of the most common causes leading to the left ventricle not pumping well enough to move the blood from the heart and into the circulatory system. Coronary artery disease can lead to a heart attack which, if the person survives, damages the heart muscle and leaves a scar. This damage reduces the heart's functional capacity, particularly if it is a large scar.

If the muscle is still alive but not receiving enough blood, it is called **viable** heart muscle. A lack of blood supply means that the muscle receives inadequate oxygen and nutrients, and cramps, affecting the way the heart contracts. Amazingly, it can appear to not function, lying 'dormant'; then, with the restoration of blood flow, it can start to function normally, again.

This is called **hibernating myocardium.**

As it is not receiving the oxygen and the nutrients it needs to function correctly, it 'cramps' in the region not receiving adequate flow. Two things happen:

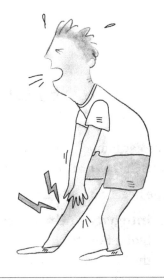

- there can be **pain**, like cramp pain, but not always, and

- the area of the heart receiving inadequate blood **becomes stiff,** which affects its ability to relax, which impacts

How long can the heart 'hibernate' like this? It's a bit like what happens when you get a cramp in a leg, say, after intense exercising when the muscles fatigue and the nutrients needed for recovery are not getting there.

on how well the main pump, the left ventricle, works. The restricted left ventricle does not relax as it should, and so does not accommodate as much blood as it should, that is, as much blood as is needed for the body's cardiac output. Thus, the blood, which should be flowing 'forward' into the left ventricle, backs up into the left atrium and even into the lungs. This increased pressure, particularly in the lungs, causes shortness of breath. This stiffness of the heart is also called a failure of relaxation or **diastolic dysfunction.** (Remember diastolic blood pressure is the pressure during the time the heart is **not** pumping, the relaxation phase.)

This is a fascinating situation. One would guess that the 'work' the heart does is in contracting. However, the energy used by the heart is for relaxation. Think of stretching and letting go of a rubber band. When triggered, the heart contracts by the interaction of proteins that draw together, recoiling like a rubber band. The stretch (relaxation) is what requires energy. The extreme example of this is rigor mortis. In this state the muscles become stiff, not flaccid, with death.

Toxic changes can also affect the function of the heart. Use of **recreational drugs** such as cocaine, and even anabolic steroids, can harm the heart muscle. Importantly, and without question most commonly, excessive **alcohol** can cause damage. Years of alcohol abuse through long-term heavy drinking and binge drinking can weaken the heart muscle. The condition most significantly affects men aged between 35 and 50 years old, but also women. Often, there are no symptoms until CF occurs.

Different **metals** can also cause damage. For example, too much copper, lead, cobalt, and even too much or too little iron can impact the way the left and right ventricles work and, therefore, the pump action of the heart.

Medications can also be toxic directly to the heart muscle. Some cancer drugs (chemotherapeutic agents), as well as anti-depressants, anti-psychotics and immune-modulating drugs, need watching. The agents used for treating cancer, which kill or manage the cancer cells, are monitored very carefully, as they can have a detrimental effect on the way the heart muscle works. **Radiation**, especially of the chest that may include direct exposure to the heart, also needs close monitoring.

Inflammation can be triggered by **infections**, which can cause problems for the heart muscle. They can be from bacteria, viruses and, in some parts of the world, parasites.

....

A parasitic infection called Chagas disease can cause altered, diminished or worsening function of the heart muscle and so lead to cardiac failure. It is a common cause of cardiac failure in South America. Chagas disease is treatable, especially if diagnosed early. Therapy is highly effective if given during the acute phase of the disease and less effective when administered during the chronic phase. Currently, two antiparasitic agents are used to treat Chagas disease, the drugs benznidazole and nifurtimox.

....

Autoimmune disorders can also cause inflammation. In such instances, the body's immune system, for whatever reason, works against itself. Conditions include rheumatoid arthritis and systemic lupus erythematosus (SLE).

Another situation that impacts how the left ventricle works is the **infiltration** of substances into the myocardium, the muscular middle layer of the wall of the heart. This intrusion can come from malignant cells from the esophagus or lungs and, sometimes, from other organs, directly accessing the heart.

On occasions, deposits of a group of proteins, the **amyloid proteins**, are found. These deposits generally are a consequence of metabolic processes going wrong, either within the liver or the bone marrow. When excess specific proteins are deposited into the left ventricle, they locate between the muscle cells, stopping the cells from functioning properly. The heart becomes stiff. As it cannot relax appropriately, it pumps less blood into the body. This is a diastolic failure.

The build-up of amyloid proteins is very hard to treat. However, recently-developed treatments for specific forms of heart-based amyloidosis offer promise.

The trick here for medicos is to remember to look for amyloid proteins, as the build-up is rarely immediately apparent.

You can choose your friends but not your **family** and that means that inherited dilated cardiomyopathy can run in families. These families have changes in the protein structure of the myofibril, the contracting component of the muscle cell. Many variations produce minor and major changes in protein structure that lead to expression (the time the condition becomes apparent in the individual) being early or late in life and, of course, with variances in severity.

Other genetic conditions – in which too much fat or too much glycogen (sugar) has been deposited in the muscle because it has not been dealt with appropriately by the body's metabolism – can cause difficulties. For example, in the inherited conditions of Gaucher disease and Fabry disease, the sufferer has a defective enzyme that leads to deranged metabolism, with the formation of by-products that are either fat-based or glucose-based. These by-products, not dealt with as part of a healthy metabolism, can accumulate within the body's tissues. Such accumulation is called a 'storage disease', which results in **infiltrative cardiomyopathy**. By-products infiltrate the heart tissues causing derangement of the tissue and loss of function.

Lastly, there is also a genetic group of mechanisms that, as the person develops and expresses that genetic disposition, can lead to the heart being too thick which then progresses to a stiff heart and cardiac failure. This condition is called **hypertrophic cardiomyopathy.** The heart is also one of the organs that can be affected by a group of inherited conditions, **muscular dystrophies,** in which the body's voluntary muscles weaken.

Other **metabolic** problems, not necessarily genetic, that can directly affect the myocardium include:

- the **thyroid** not working properly;

- **calcium levels** being too high or too low;

- **growth hormone** abnormality;

- **nutritional** issues, such as lack of vitamin B1 (thiamine) or arising from multi-factorial problems from malnutrition, mal-absorption and iron deficiency.

The build-up of proteins, fats, or glycogen are very specific conditions needing specialized intervention.

CASE STUDY – BARNEY

shortness of breath, HFrEF, left bundle
branch block, amyloidosis

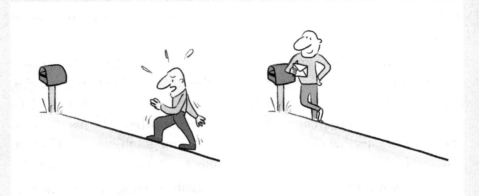

Barney was a fit 81-year-old when we met. His wife accompanied him to the consultation. He was generally well, although he had had minor medical issues including a pulmonary embolism (PE) in association with orthopedic surgery. PE is a well-recognized complication and had been well managed. Mostly, he was well and active until several months before coming to see me. During those months, he had described to his local doctor shortness of breath that was apparent walking to the letterbox and undertaking general tasks around the house. The letterbox was an excellent example because there was a small incline to reach it.

Barney looked in good shape, physically. He was not carrying excess weight. He didn't have high blood pressure, nor did he have elevated cholesterol levels. While his ECG showed normal sinus rhythm, it also showed a left bundle branch block, which meant that the electrical impulses that activate the heart muscle were passing through the heart in a slightly discordant way. The bundles of Purkinje fibres (like copper wires) that distribute the electricity through the heart were not functioning correctly.

The electrical signal had to propagate through the muscle itself, muscle cell to next muscle cell, rather than through the 'wires' as normal to distribute the electrical signal throughout the muscle. A chest x-ray, organized by his GP to investigate Barney's shortness of breath, had shown features of fluid on the lungs, suggesting cardiac failure.

Barney was then referred to me for evaluation. An ultrasound, used to obtain an assessment of how the heart was performing, showed diminished function. Left bundle branch block generally produces a reduction of the heart's coordination, reducing its efficiency. Barney's ejection fraction was 40 percent, and probably in keeping with the electrical abnormality. What was notable, though, was that the walls of the ventricle appeared to be thickened and speckled. These characteristics raised the possibility of an infiltrative process. When we did our measurements, looking at flow patterns and the way the heart relaxed, these patterns also confirmed that the heart was quite stiff.

The heart, because it is stiff, does not relax properly and so diastolic failure occurs (diastolic meaning the relaxation phase of the heart function). This is quite significant.

Barney's ultrasound results suggested an infiltrative process in which a protein, called amyloid protein, finds its way into the heart muscle, thickens it, makes it stiff and shows a characteristic speckled appearance. We investigated for amyloidosis by undertaking a bone marrow test and a nuclear medicine scan.

The bone marrow test was organized because cancer cells within the bone marrow can sometimes produce proteins which form amyloid proteins, and those amyloid proteins can then congregate in the heart, making it stiff. So, Barney underwent a bone marrow investigation. There was no problem. That the bone marrow was clear was reassuring that there wasn't an underlying cancer or nasty infective or inflammatory process driving these changes in his heart.

Barney also underwent a nuclear medicine scan, a particular study that uses an isotope (a radioactive tracer detectable by a gamma camera) that attaches to the searched-for protein. His heart lit up like a Christmas tree, thus confirming a diagnosis of amyloidosis. Barney had senile amyloidosis or amyloidosis of the elderly. Generally, this form has a far more benign and gradual prognosis than other types of amyloidosis.

I treated Barney's cardiac failure (even though he had preserved ejection fraction) with a beta-blocker, bisoprolol, an ACE inhibitor, ramipril, and spironolactone. When Barney came back to see me a few weeks later, however, he just didn't want to admit that he was feeling better. He wanted to spend all his time in the consultation complaining about taking medications. It was only when I asked his wife for some input that she said, quite freely, that he was walking up to the letterbox without any problems at all.

Barney eventually agreed that he was feeling substantially better. He wanted to complain about taking tablets because he didn't like doing it. Barney had

It can be very valuable to have another person present to offer objective information.

lived for 80-plus years without having taken any tablets. Why should he want to start now?

His reluctance opened up an opportunity for a sensible discussion about the pros and cons of taking medication: risk and benefit. For Barney, the risk from taking the tablets was pretty small, and the tablets were working well. The benefit was evident, in his walking to the letterbox. After a discussion, Barney, with the support of his wife, realized that the medications were doing the job. He remains on those. We have added a small amount of the diuretic, furosemide, to be taken on an as-needed basis if fluid accumulates in his body, maybe a couple of tablets, occasionally, and no more than a few times a week.

When I last saw Barney, he was in good fettle, and I am looking forward to seeing him in another six months.

abnormal loading of the heart

Another group of causes of heart failure relates to abnormal loading of the heart, which means there is a **pressure** problem that results in cardiac failure. The most common is elevated **blood pressure** (hypertension).

Increased pressure in the circulation directly affects the workload of the heart. Long-standing raised blood pressure causes physical changes to the heart in order to deal with the increased load. To help it work harder, the heart thickens. That makes it stiff, which means it does not relax properly, and, therefore, does not pump properly. In this diastolic failure, stiff hearts fail at the time the heart should be relaxing.

Think of working your bicep muscle in the gym. The muscle thickens in response to the load or training. This is good for your bicep, but not so good for your heart.

The wear and tear on **heart valves** cause other significant issues. Valves can be tight and affect 'forward' flow, or they can leak and allow the blood to flow 'backwards' in the wrong direction.

Imagine that the aortic valve is too **narrow**. The left ventricle needs to pump harder with increased pressure to move the blood out of the heart and into the body. The result is similar to the person having high blood pressure.

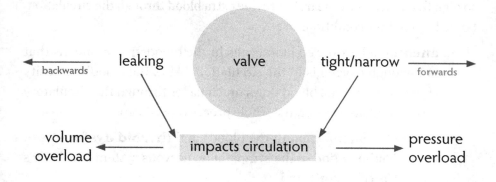

when a valve does not work

What if the valve **leaks**, so that every time the ventricle pumps blood out, some leaks back in, lessening the amount of blood pumped around the body? The heart tries to accommodate by dilating the left ventricle, increasing its size so that it pumps an increased volume of blood into the circulation. While some of the blood regurgitates into the left ventricle, enough is pumped into the circulatory system to meet the body's requirements.

Should any one of the heart's valves – the aortic, the mitral, the pulmonary or the tricuspid valve – have a problem, such as being tight and limiting forward flow, or leaking and allowing reverse flow, it has an impact on the circulation. In the forward direction, it affects pressure while in the reverse direction, it increases volume and causes congestion.

Think of an overcoat becoming a straitjacket

The outside of the heart has a covering called the **pericardium** (*peri*, around; *cardium*, heart). If this thickens, it acts as a constricting cover around the heart, limiting relaxation of the muscle and leading to heart failure. The interior surface of the heart's chambers also has a special lining, the **endocardium** (*endo*, inner; *cardium*, heart). It, too, can be affected by disease. If it thickens and stiffens, this also affects how the heart relaxes and can give rise to cardiac failure.

If the body requires a large amount of cardiac output, then the system can be overloaded. **High output failure** occurs when the body's requirement is so high that it drives the heart to provide extra blood through the circulation. Some high output conditions are:

- **anemia**, a lack of red blood cells in the bloodstream, means that not enough oxygen is in the circulation. Also, the blood's viscosity changes so that the blood flows much faster through the circulatory system and, as a result, the whole process speeds up.

- **sepsis** (a bad infection in the blood) and **thyroid dysfunction**, through stimulation of the sympathetic nervous system (the body's natural 'accelerator'), and

- **Paget's disease of bone** where the bones become hyper-metabolic, meaning there is marked increase in formation and absorption of bone, albeit deranged, and so the demand for blood increases.

> *High output is like revving the engine of a car into the red zone for extended periods. Revving is not good for the engine, nor is high output good for your heart.*

Additional load can be put on the system by **increased fluid**. Let's say, five or six liters of blood flow around the body at a given time. If this were increased fairly quickly to 7-10 liters, in a closed system, the fluid needs to go somewhere, and so increased pressure is felt throughout the whole system: the right side of the heart, the lungs and the left side of the heart.

Such fluid accumulation can occur if the kidneys suddenly are not functioning correctly. Urine is not produced and, so, the body is not letting go of the fluid. Another setting is patients in hospitals. Patients can be given fluids during surgery or in relation to their illness. Sometimes they can be given too much fluid, creating an iatrogenic (*iatro,* physician or medical treatment; *genic,* producing or causing) situation. Rest assured that medical carers monitor fluid levels closely, as they are aware of the dangers of fluid overload.

abnormal timing

The speed of the heartbeat is the third element in considering the causes of cardiac failure. A heart beating too fast or too slow creates problems.

If the heartbeat is too **fast**, one of the high output states described above could be driving it, or the heart's electrical system could be **faulty**. One of the most common settings of the heart's electrical system driving the heart rate too fast is **atrial fibrillation** (AF). If the heart rate is rapid and poorly controlled, the rate can race at well over 100 beats per minute for a prolonged period. The heart can decompensate and go into failure.

If the heart beats **too slowly**, the cardiac output for the person is not enough, and can result in decreased energy, shortness of breath and even blackout. And the heart can fail, also.

IMPORTANT POINTS

There are three main pathways to cardiac failure:

- the muscle
- heart load
- heart rate.

However, the usual suspects are:

- coronary artery disease
  - scarring
  - lack of blood flow / diastolic dysfunction
- toxicity
- alcohol
- hypertension (particularly significant if the heart appears to have a normal structure and pumps well but does not relax well)
- atrial fibrillation
- fluid overload (particularly in renal failure).

If the primary cause can be determined, it opens up the possibility of treatment.

CASE STUDY – FREDDY

shortness of breath, earlier heart problems, dilated left atrium, HFpEF, marginal pulmonary pressures, hard-to-demonstrate fluid retention

Although I knew Freddy for years in the community in which I live, he was 72 years old when he first came to see me with shortness of breath. Earlier in his life, he had played numerous sports at a very high level, and he still lived an active life. When he came to see me, he was swimming regularly, spent a lot of time on his stationary bike, and he loved to travel.

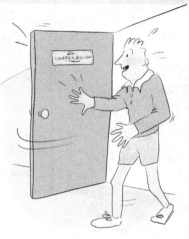

"Warrick, you're a bloody magician!"

Five years earlier, in his mid-to-late 60s, he had required a pacemaker because of heart rhythm disturbance. With that implantation, he returned to normal function quickly, and the pacemaker was working well. Two years before the pacemaker implant, in his early-to-mid 60s, he had suffered from chest pain, which proved to be a tight blockage of the artery running down the front of his heart. The artery, the left anterior descending, is the one nearest to the chest wall. The implantation of a stent resolved the problem. A stress test, when he presented with the shortness of breath (as it may have been a manifestation of lack of blood flow to the heart), did not show any problems with his blood flow, giving some reassurance that the stent was working well.

We can see a dilated left atrium as people age, and, certainly, it can be related to elevated blood pressure over the years.

At the same time, we undertook an echocardiogram to look at how Freddy's heart was working. While the left ventricle, the main pumping chamber, was pumping well, the left atrium, the pre-pump chamber on the left side, was a little dilated.

His pulmonary pressures were marginal. A measured pulmonary pressure of around 30-35 millimeters of mercury was high enough for me to think perhaps that, in the absence of lack of blood flow being an issue for Freddy, retention of fluid could be a problem. Retention of fluid can sometimes be hard to demonstrate.

If someone has severe cardiac failure, we see clear features of fluid retention

- *while sitting across from a patient, the neck veins are prominent due to the extra fluid in the circulation*

- *ankles are swollen*

- *a distinct sock line is obvious*

- *mention could be made of not being able to get feet into shoes.*

These are indicators that there is too much fluid in the circulatory system. These people with the above clear physical features show clear biochemical markers, too. If we were to measure indicators of cardiac failure, such as brain natriuretic peptide levels, they would register at the high end of the range or be clearly into the range demonstrating cardiac failure. In some patients, it's just not as obvious. Thus, for some patients with heart failure in the setting of preserved ejection fraction, the signs can be very subtle and quite difficult to pin down.

With that in mind, and for several other reasons — Freddy's age, his pre-diabetic status, history of elevated blood pressure (although now treated), known ischemia and therefore some wear and tear on the heart and the vasculature — I thought there was a chance that Freddy had heart failure with preserved ejection fraction.

I gave Freddy a diagnostic trial of diuretic therapy. I prescribed him the loop diuretic, furosemide, with the instructions to take one or two tablets, depending on his symptoms, for no more than three days in a seven-day week.

Well, Freddy took the instructions on board and off he went. He returned some six to eight weeks later. Waltzing through the door, he exclaimed, "Warrick, you're a bloody magician!" So, I didn't have to ask how he was.

Freddy was a fantastic example of someone with preserved ejection fraction, with some retention of fluid that was difficult to clearly demonstrate. A diagnostic trial of fluid tablets made a difference.

Sometimes when the diagnosis is not clear-cut, a medication is prescribed in the hope that it will make a difference. This is a diagnostic trial. If the use of the medication confirms the diagnosis, then the drug is continued in order to maintain the therapeutic benefit.

Armed with that regime, Freddy went on for several years popping a fluid tablet as needed. I continued to keep a close eye on his cholesterol levels, making sure he was on target, and on his blood pressure. I interrogated his pacemaker regularly, and we mitigated his risk of diabetes by keeping a close eye on exercise and lifestyle.

While Freddy proved to be an appreciative patient, he was also a great patient, taking on board all the advice and medication I offered. With proper management around the issues regarding his cardiovascular health, he was able to pursue a full and active life.

I'm really sad to say that Freddy has since died. It was not his heart that caused his death. Five years after I saw him for his shortness of breath, he was traveling and enjoying life to the max when he had an unfortunate accident that took him from us.

RIP, Freddy. You are missed.

With all its complexities,
how is cardiac failure diagnosed?

chapter 7
DIAGNOSIS AND INVESTIGATION

Cardiac failure requires a clinical diagnosis. This begins with taking the patient's history and performing a medical examination. The two symptoms the patients are most likely to present with are **shortness of breath** and **swelling**.

shortness of breath

In considering shortness of breath as a symptom, (occasionally accompanied by a cough), there are three considerations:

- **timing.** If it comes on rapidly, it is called **acute**; if it comes on gradually, it is called **chronic**.

- **intensity.** The New York Heart Association (NYHA) classification of cardiac failure refers to four levels of intensity, with four described as shortness of breath with minimal exertion, almost at rest; one described as almost negligible shortness of breath at extremes of exercise; and levels two and three sitting between these extremes. *(refer to the table on page 102)*

- **position.** If patients with cardiac failure lie down, there can be shifts of fluid within the body; for example, fluid moves towards the lungs whilst lying, and the fluid drains away into the legs when the person stands up. Shortness of breath in the supine position is known as orthopnea. In contrast, frightening shortness of breath that wakes the person up in the middle of the night is **p**aroxysmal (intermittent) **n**octurnal (night-time) **d**ysphonia (shortness of breath) or PND.

New York Heart Association (NYHA) Classification of Cardiac Failure	
class I (mild)	No limitation of physical activity. Ordinary physical activity does not cause undue breathlessness, fatigue or palpitations.
class II (mild)	Slight limitation of physical activity. Comfortable at rest, but ordinary physical activity results in undue breathlessness, fatigue or palpitations.
class III (moderate)	Marked limitation of physical activity. Comfortable at rest, but less than ordinary physical activity results in undue breathlessness, fatigue or palpitations.
class IV (severe)	Unable to perform any physical activity without discomfort. Symptoms can be present at rest. Physical activity increases discomfort.

swelling

Knowledge of the patient's history of swelling is also important. Patients will have noticed if their legs have been swollen like balloons. However, information about more subtle swelling is also significant. Has a patient seen significant 'sock marks' where, over time, their socks have made an indentation into their ankles? Fluid in the legs is called **peripheral edema** (*peripheral*, arms and legs; *edema*, swelling).

Swelling is particularly informative if it is present during the consultation. We can press our thumb into the shinbone. If a divot forms where the fluid is displaced, it clearly shows the presence of unwanted water.

other information

Medical history, especially about childhood health issues, is also essential.

- Was there a childhood murmur (a heart sound caused by turbulent blood flow through a heart valve)?

- Was there childhood cardiac or lung surgery?

- Were there fevers or infections, such a rheumatic fever, that might have impacted the person at a young age, or is there a family history of heart problems?

- Has there been a heart attack in the past?

- What's the history of blood pressure?

- Is that person short of breath at rest?

When we examine the patient, we also look for clues about how the body is responding to cardiac failure.

  - was the person breathless while walking into the consulting room, getting into or out of a chair, or getting undressed?

- What is the pulse rate?

  - is it going fast, and how regular is it?

  - is it 'irregularly irregular', pointing to atrial fibrillation (AF), which can be associated with heart failure?

- Is the blood pressure very high?

  - could this be a driver towards heart failure?

- Is the blood pressure very low?

  - the possible implication here is that the heart is weak. The blood vessels of the body dilate, and the pressures are low because the heart is not working optimally.

Typically, doctors look at the patient's **neck**, in particular, at the venous wave, the pulsation of the skin seen from the movement of the underlying vessel, in this case, the jugular vein. Remember the large veins, the inferior vena cava (IVC) and the superior vena cava (SVC)? The SVC is one of the major veins in the body and carries blood from the top of the body to the heart. The jugular vein that carries blood from the brain, face and neck, connects with the SVC to take the blood to the right atrium. Because this fluid all 'connects', the jugular vein is like a dipstick for telling the doctor about the fluid pressure in the right atrium.

In CF, the pressures in the right atrium can be increased, and so the waveform of the jugular pulse is often visible in patients when sitting upright. The jugular pulse is not apparent in a sitting patient with a healthy heart.

It takes a bit of practice to learn how to assess the jugular venous pulse (JVP), but it is a skill worth learning for medicos. Some humor can creep into the moment. Often, patients feel a bit uneasy if they think I am staring intently at their necks. Weird! I do, of course, explain. The other thing that makes me laugh is my heart failure patients seem to have an infinite array of polo neck jumpers; so, I can't see a thing! A quick pull of the collar to one side and all is good.

Then we listen to the **heart**.

Although we are listening for normal heartbeats, we also listen for:

- various indications that tell us how a valve is working, and if it's not, then how severe the dysfunction might be

  - a blowing murmur or a rumbling murmur,

  - murmurs that get louder,

  - murmurs that get softer or

  - murmurs that get louder and softer;

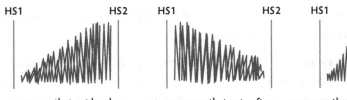

heart sounds

- extra sounds related to how the blood is filling the ventricle. As blood flows into the left ventricle it can make a noise as it hits the wall of the chamber;

- a third heart sound heard during mid-diastole that suggests a big 'baggy' heart, and

- a fourth heart sound heard just before systole that suggests the heart is thick and stiff.

After the heart, we listen to the **lungs.**

We listen specifically for evidence of fluid accumulation, which is indicated by a noise heard near the bottom of the lungs near the diaphragm. As the person breathes in, there are fine, crackly sounds called **crepitations.** Think, gentle scrunching of cellophane. These noises can represent fluid within the tissues of the lungs and also indicate severity. The more noise, the worse is the condition. If this resolves with treatment, then it is a good sign.

Understanding the significance of the noises and documenting them well is important.

We will often also examine the **abdomen**.

If heart failure, particularly right heart failure, has been present for some time, then the congestion may have caused swelling in the legs and also swelling of the organs of the abdomen, such as the liver. Occasionally, fluid can also accumulate in the tummy, making the person appear distended. Fluid in the abdomen is called **ascites**. We detect this by listening to the sound made from tapping on the tummy, rolling the patient and tapping again. A change in the pitch indicates that the fluid level has changed; 'shifting dullness'.

As part of a standard assessment for someone presenting with shortness of breath where we suspect cardiac failure, we also investigate using a 12-lead **electrocardiogram (ECG).**

This often-used test provides a great deal of information about the heart:

- how fast is the heart beating?
- is it rapid or too slow?
- is the rhythm normal?
- has it gone out of rhythm or
- is it under strain?

The QRS complex, the 'spiky bits' on the ECG readout, can provide some clues. If these are exaggerated, or large, then the heart is under some strain, indicating that the muscle has thickened or dilated as it has tried to accommodate the extra load.

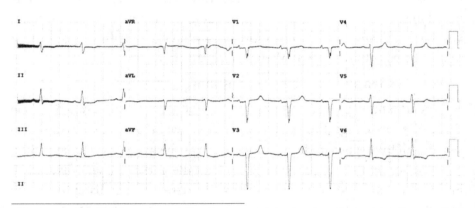

an ECG trace that shows a heart under strain

We also take a **chest x-ray** to learn the size of the heart and if fine features called **Kerley B lines** are present.

Kerley B lines are little lines within the lungs as seen on the x-ray that correspond to the crepitations (remember the crunching cellophane?) we hear when someone is suffering cardiac failure.

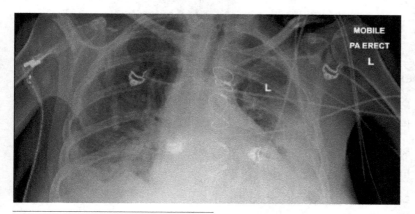

an x-ray showing Kerley B lines

Lastly, as part of a routine assessment, we would do some **blood work**, investigating normal biochemistry. We would check that

- the electrolyte levels (sodium-potassium balance) are normal;
- the kidneys are functioning well;
- no infection could be driving the process, and
- the liver function is okay.

We would also check for

- anemia,
- thyroid function, and
- iron levels

to ensure there were no obvious reversible drivers or other underlying causes to the symptoms with which the patient has presented.

Should there be congestion, it is important to check that the liver is working correctly.

107

In the early stages of assessment

- always start with a history
  - shortness of breath
  - swelling
- then look for signs or clues
  - pulse
  - JVP
  - heart sounds
  - lung sounds
  - abdomen and peripheral edema
- and then undertake tests to obtain more information
  - electrocardiogram (ECG)
  - chest x-ray
  - bloods

This chapter has presented some of the basic tests undertaken when cardiac failure is suspected in a patient. In the next chapter, we look at tests particular to cardiac failure.

chapter 8
MORE SPECIFIC TESTS

With indications pointing to cardiac failure as the problem, how do we discover what's going on with someone's heart? There are several tests available that are very specific to CF: echocardiogram, B-type natriuretic peptide, treadmill or stress testing, various cardiac imaging techniques, and biopsy.

echocardiogram

The single most important test is an ultrasound of the heart, an echocardiogram (*echo*, sound; *cardio,* heart; *ography*, picture). An **'echo'** provides a fantastic, real-time, dynamic study that looks at how the heart functions with each beat. It shows

- how the muscle is contracting and relaxing (helping evaluate diastolic function);
- the right side of the heart;
- the left side;
- the atria, and
- the ventricles.

Also,

- chambers can be evaluated together or independently;
- size can be compared;
- function, which includes how well the heart is contracting but also, importantly, how well it is relaxing, can be assessed, and
- it also shows how much blood the left ventricle is expelling with each beat. As we have already seen, the amount of blood expelled, expressed as a percentage of the total volume of the left ventricle, is the ejection fraction, a significant figure in starting to understand what's going on within that individual.

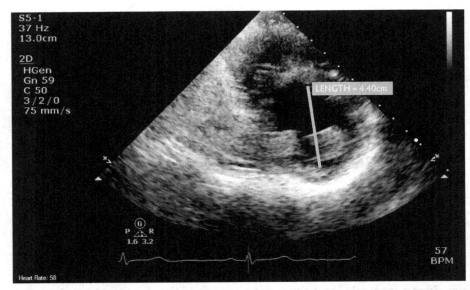

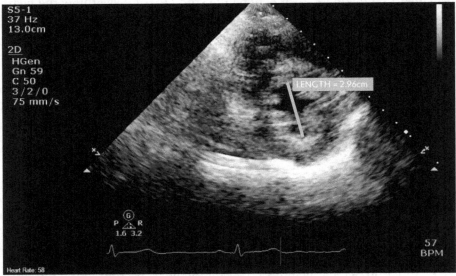

An echocardiogram, or ultrasound, or 'echo' of the heart, shows heart structure and valves. This is a healthy heart: diastole (top) and systole.

If there is a problem, the echocardiogram shows if the entire heart has been affected equally. If all of the heart has been affected, it is called a **global** abnormality. If only a part of the heart is not working, it is called a **regional** abnormality.

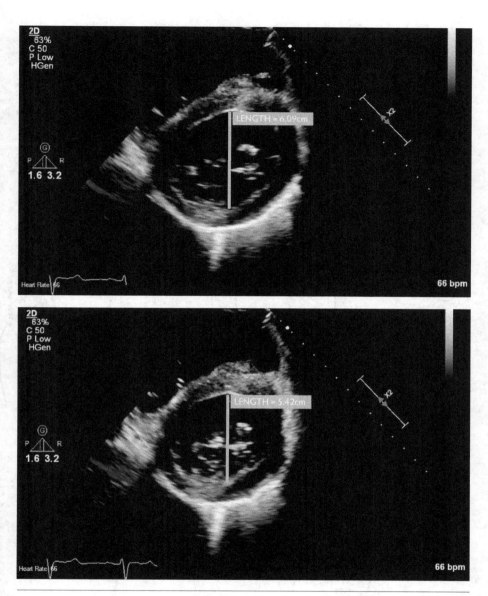

This is a dilated heart in cardiac failure: diastole (top) and systole.

For example, when a blocked blood vessel gives rise to myocardial infarction (heart attack) that leaves scar tissue where the muscle, starved of blood, has died. This is a regional problem.

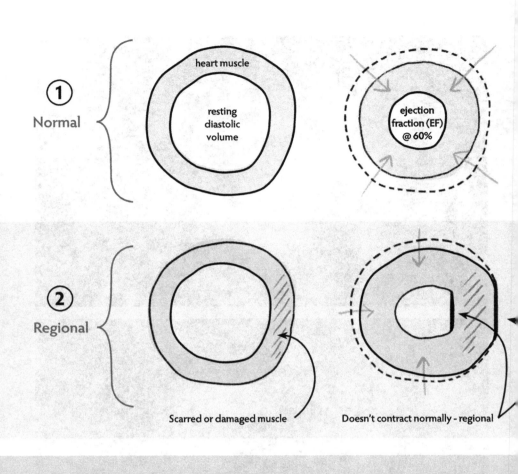

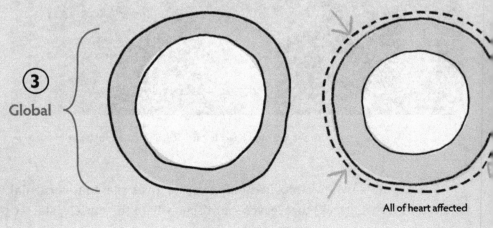

① **Normal**

heart muscle

resting diastolic volume

ejection fraction (EF) @ 60%

② **Regional**

Scarred or damaged muscle

Doesn't contract normally - regional

③ **Global**

All of heart affected

global or regional?

An echocardiogram is also extremely valuable for looking at the **valves**. The working capacity of each valve can be assessed individually. Determining flow through the valves helps ascertain pressures within the heart and the valves, themselves. Velocity assessment (that is relating velocity to pressure) is used to calculate pressures within the heart and this, too, becomes vital data.

This information is the beginning of making plans.

An echocardiogram is an invaluable tool that has completely revolutionized the way we can deal with cardiac failure and guide therapy.

b-type natriuretic peptide

B-type **n**atriuretic **p**eptide (BNP, also known as **brain n**atriuretic **p**eptide) is particularly useful if the cardiologist thinks that there *could* be a problem with the heart, but is still unsure. The test is a very beneficial discriminator to help clarify if there is a problem with the heart or if the shortness of breath is related to something other than the heart.

BNP is a substance released by the heart cells when they are under strain. It is part of the natriuretic peptide system. If a patient is short of breath and the heart is working well, BNP is normal. However, if it's not, then there is a strain within the heart and it requires further investigation.

In the longer term, its use is valuable when reviewing patients who have a valve abnormality, as it can be used regularly in association with an ultrasound to check the problem valve.

- If the echocardiogram shows the valve getting worse and the BNP increases, then we can be pretty sure that things are worsening for that patient.

- If the echocardiogram looks unchanged, yet the BNP has increased, the heart may be under more strain than is being shown by the echocardiogram. Further investigation is warranted.

- If the echocardiogram suggests worsening changes in the valve, yet the BNP has not changed, that invites the cardiologist to look more closely again at the echocardiogram.

treadmill or stress testing

Stress testing may be considered appropriate for patients who can exercise. If necessary, drugs are available that can replicate exercise and, so, the heart assessment can occur without the patient having to exercise at all. This drug-based test is a **pharmacological** stress test.

Stress testing is used mainly to evaluate:

- blood flow to the heart;
- exercise capacity, and
- symptoms.

other cardiac imaging

Direct evaluation for coronary artery disease may include

- **CT imaging** of the heart to assess the health of the arteries in a non-invasive way, or
- **invasive angiography**, where a catheter (thin tube) is directed into the heart arteries so that dye may be injected into the arteries to obtain a very clear picture of the narrowings of the arteries.

Ascertaining if coronary artery disease is contributing to an individual's cardiac dysfunction is important as, in many situations, remedial action is available.

Magnetic **R**esonance **I**maging (MRI) is an imaging technique that uses huge magnets to excite water particles in the tissues in a way that generates a picture. When used in relation to the heart, it is called **cardiac magnetic resonance** (CMR). An exquisite test, it produces beautiful images. It is incredibly valuable in showing scarring within the heart, and inflammation. So, if someone's left ventricle is not working correctly, CMR can reveal inflammation, the integrity of the cells and the presence/absence of scar tissue, thus giving information related to the muscle and the connective tissue. A CMR also shows heart function and valve function superbly well and provides information on regurgitation, leaking valves and narrowing of valves. This information is significant in determining a future management plan for any individual with CF.

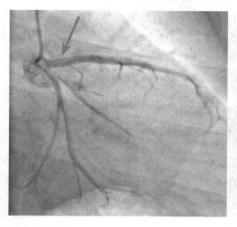

invasive angiogram

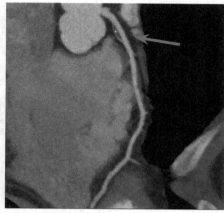

CT angiogram

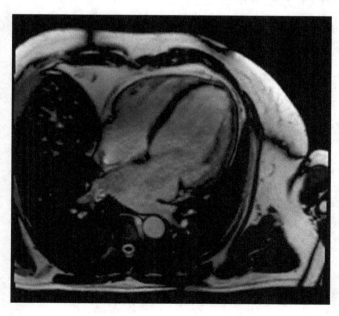

cardiac magnetic resonance

biopsy

Finally, and rarely, if further information is *still* needed, a biopsy is performed. This is significant. It is not performed everywhere, and it is certainly not a routine test. However, occasionally, a small piece of heart muscle tissue is put under a microscope to see what is occurring at the cellular level. It may confirm an infiltrative process, such as amyloid proteins, or it could show inflammatory cells, for example, in the setting of myocarditis, which is inflammation of the myocardium (heart muscle).

IMPORTANT POINTS

Specific cardiac failure testing includes

- **echocardiogram**, the workhorse test of cardiac failure assessment

- **B-type natriuretic peptide** measurement

- **stress testing**, either on a machine or, occasionally, with drugs if the patient cannot exercise

- non-invasive or invasive **coronary imaging,** to determine the health of the coronary arteries

- cardiac magnetic resonance **(CMR) imaging** to give more information

- **biopsy,** a possible, but not standard, test

With a cardiac failure diagnosis confirmed, what do we do about it?

THE HEART
CARDIAC FAILURE TREATMENT

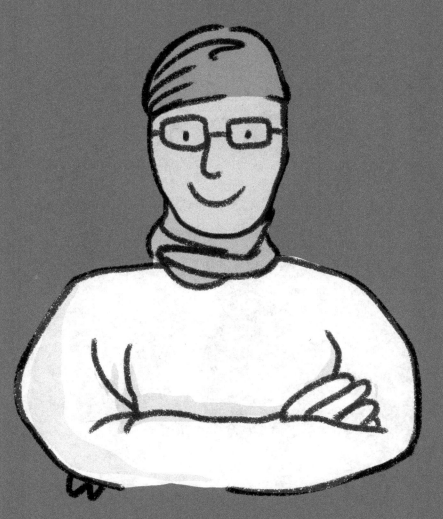

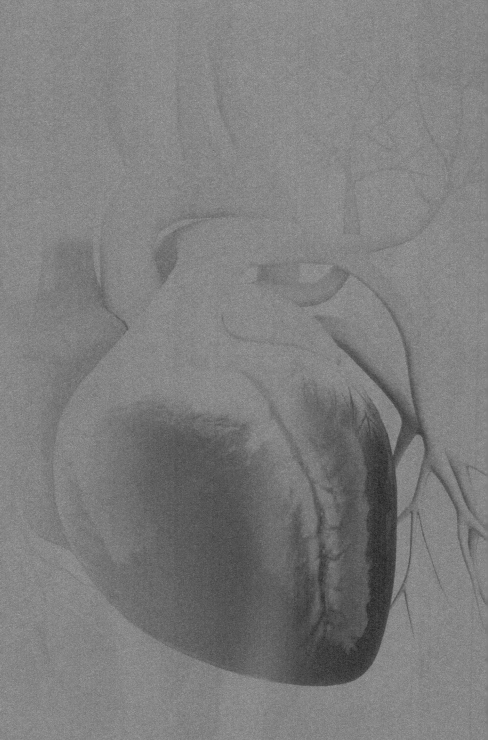

CASE STUDY – KATHLEEN

shortness of breath, NYHA 4, HFpEF, one kidney, low glomerular filtration rate

Kathleen was a 'young' 98-year-old when I first met her. Her general practitioner had sent her to me because she was suffering from shortness of breath and was classified as New York Heart Association 4, meaning that she had shortness of breath with minimal or no exertion. Kathleen was living independently, was intellectually sound and enjoying life. She particularly enjoyed a glass of pinot noir with dinner. Kathleen had been in good health and active for most of her life. She had donated a kidney to a family member, which meant that she was in close contact with a renal doctor, or nephrologist, to ensure that her remaining kidney was cared for well.

If you are functioning with one kidney, you need to look after it.

Kathleen's GP had realized that the shortness of breath with associated swelling of the legs was likely to be related to how the heart was functioning and had, quite reasonably, started diuretic therapy to draw fluid out of her body. The doctor had also prescribed Kathleen an ACE inhibitor to offset some of the issues related to heart failure. By providing some vasodilation (dilation of the blood vessels), blood pressure decreased and the environment in which the heart worked was improved.

When I saw Kathleen, the problem was that her health was alternating between decreased renal function and shortness of breath. Diuretic therapy caused a decrease in the renal function; the shortness of breath returned when the diuretic therapy was removed. So, when she was 'dried out', her shortness of breath was improved, but the kidney was deteriorating. Yet, when the diuretic therapy was stopped to allow the kidney to recover, the shortness of breath came back. This was a trouble, as neither shortness of breath nor a poorly-functioning kidney is desirable, the latter especially so as Kathleen had only the one kidney.

An ultrasound of Kathleen's heart demonstrated that Kathleen was suffering heart failure with preserved ejection fraction, HFpEF. Although she had a stiff heart, it was contracting well. Her glomerular filtration rate was 35. This rate is a measure of how well the kidneys are filtering the blood and is an approximation of urine production. Preferably, this should be 60 or above, so 35 was compromised.

When I first saw Kathleen, her symptoms were not too bad. She had been on diuretic therapy, so her kidney function was down. What we needed was a regime that would walk the fine line between her body being too dry and too wet, so that we could maintain the kidney function yet minimize the breathlessness. Based on the clinical assessment and her renal function at the time, it was likely that Kathleen was a little too dry.

It is quite common that as people age, the heart becomes stiffer.

We decided to use her body weight as a marker for fluid retention. I put to her that I thought her ideal weight was a kilogram heavier than what it was on the day when I saw her, that is, I thought she needed an extra liter of fluid 'on board'. So, we created 57 kg as a set-point, her 'ideal' weight.

The idea was that if her weight dropped below that ideal weight, she would not take any diuretic therapy as there was no point in taking fluid off if the fluid balance was good. Then, I gave Kathleen a sliding-scale, take-as-needed, regime for her diuretic therapy. If, for example, Kathleen went a kilogram **above** her ideal weight, she would use a certain amount of her diuretic therapy to bring her weight back to the ideal by passing off the excess, retained fluid. If, somehow, she drifted to two kilograms above, she would then double her diuretic therapy and try to bring the weight back to her ideal figure.

Kathleen, and her daughter, who was with her, thought it was a good idea. When they came back two weeks later, it hadn't worked as I had hoped. Kathleen had suffered another episode of shortness of breath, and her kidney function wasn't any better.

We re-established that her ideal weight was 57 kg, and I explained the concept again in detail. I also suggested that Kathleen graph this out and keep track of it daily.

Two weeks later, Kathleen and her daughter came in, both with a spring in their steps and both absolutely delighted with Kathleen's progress. Kathleen proudly showed me the chart that she had dutifully kept, all excellently written on graph paper, exactly documenting her weight and what doses she had been taking, day-to-day. She understood that a tight bandwidth exists between too much and too little fluid. We had found the sweet spot. By adjusting her diuretic therapy based on her weight, she had been able to maintain that ideal hydration within her body. Kathleen was excited that she had some ownership and control over her diuretic therapy and her kidney function.

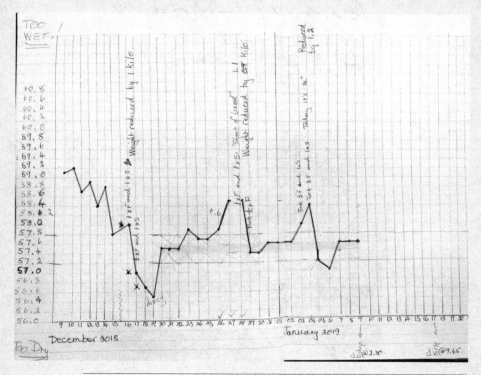

Kathleen's well-kept graph

At Kathleen's most recent visit, her glomerular filtration rate had risen from 35 to 50. This rise was nearly a 50 percent improvement in her renal function, a substantial improvement for a person with one kidney. Symptomatically, Kathleen had not had further episodes of the

Adjusting therapy doses as required is a common technique.
I use it regularly with my patients with heart failure.

shortness of breath. Her New York Heart Association classification 4 was down to a classification 2. She was still living independently, enjoying life, especially her nightly glass of pinot. She was doing a fabulous job. She had owned the problem and had worked at finding the best solution. It is now 2020, and we have celebrated her 100th birthday!

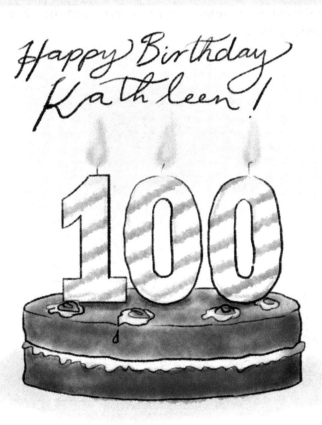

KATHLEEN'S JOURNEY

I'm 99, going well, eating well, and still here to laugh and enjoy a glass of pinot with my family and friends. I spend more time reading books now that I've slowed down, but most days I still check my plants in the greenhouse.

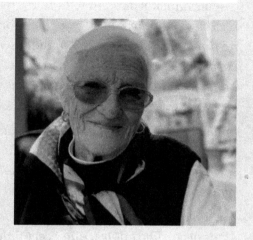

I have a special seat in the greenhouse where I rest in the warmth while sending emails to overseas friends and catching up on local gossip on my mobile. On my energetic days, I transplant my seedlings from the greenhouse to the garden.

I have always loved growing my own vegetables to feed my 10 children who now take turns to give a hand doing the heavy jobs. Tino from Gardening Australia[5] recently came to give me a hand.

He planted my zucchini, beans and cucumber seedlings that I had grown from seeds. I was a bit disappointed; the cameras should have filmed me planting not him. I don't think the team realized how well I'm doing.

Life wasn't as good two to three years ago when I started to feel breathless and had to keep opening windows to get enough oxygen. I knew I was on the way out. I felt sad and miserable but kept telling myself that at least I was fortunate to have lasted longer than my mother and husband who only made it to 94 and 93, respectively.

My energy had dropped considerably; my garden suffered. I was dragging my heels but didn't tell my children. I tried to pick myself up. I had to, there was no time to waste!

I started preparing by sorting out all my photos, books, knitted dolls, bits 'n' pieces to be given to my children, grandchildren and great-grandchildren when I departed.

One day, my daughter, Jane, arrived unexpectedly to find me with my head well out the window gasping for oxygen on a cold winter's day. In no time, she had made an appointment with my GP who referred me to a cardiologist. Why, I didn't know, as I couldn't see any connection between one's heart and ongoing breathlessness.

Straight away, my cardiologist referred me to a renal specialist, and again, I didn't know why, except that he was probably extra careful as I only have one kidney. I had donated a kidney to my son 25 years earlier. I've always perceived myself as an active, robust person, preferring a healthy plant-based diet while trying to avoid medication as much as possible.

I now know I was somewhat naïve about the situation. I had the first signs of cardiac failure. And I certainly didn't realize that my cardiologist could work a 'miracle' to restore and improve my health.

There were significant concerns about the potential adverse effect of medication on my only kidney, so my cardiologist organized regular, frequent tests to monitor and check its function. These tests were quite a process, but the adjustments to the medication gave my heart a helping hand while not affecting my kidney in the slightest.

I was amazed by this detailed process. Just a little medication made such a massive difference to how I was feeling.

Drawing a diagram, my cardiologist explained the process and the need to monitor my body's 'dry' weight and 'wet' weight. Initially, this weight business was all a bit confusing. When I started to gain too much weight, I learnt that my body was retaining fluid, and when I lost weight, I, therefore, knew I was moving towards dehydration. It was a very tricky situation, so my daughter helped me draw up a graph so that I could record my weight each morning. With advice from my cardiologist, we established the median between my dry and wet weight. This figure helped me to manage the level of medication my body needed from day-to-day.

So, now I know that when my weight increases well over the median level, my body needs a little support with the help of one furosemide. Brilliant! At first, it was so complicated. Now, the graph gives me simple visual feedback which enables me to control and participate in the process. I'm so pleased that I only to take one furosemide when needed rather than one every day.

So here I am, still living in my own home, sitting next to my favorite window, not gasping for oxygen with my head out the window! The medical professionals are fantastic. How things have changed since my birth in 1920! I really appreciate the complicated and persistent work my cardiologist has done to give my heart well-needed support. I value the richness of my life and the privilege to sit here right now as I organize the invitations for my 100th. ♥

[5] *Gardening Australia* is an Australia-wide gardening program presented by leading horticulturists on Australia's national broadcaster, the Australian Broadcasting Commission (ABC). Tino is Tino Carnevale, the Tasmanian presenter. The segment was called "Celebrating a Century" and wizard on Friday, 28 February 2020. The program can be seen on Gardening Australia, https://www.abc.net.au/gardening/factsheets/celebrating-a-century/12010706

epilogue:

Kathleen died on 25 May 2021 at 101 years young.

RIP, Kathleen. What a woman.

Cardiac failure, itself, is complex; its co-morbidities can be multi-faceted; treatment is remainder-of-life. Yet, when CF is well-treated, for many, the heart can recover, symptoms improve and the person's chance of a sudden death reduces.

chapter 9
TREATMENT – AN OVERVIEW

As we turn our attention to treatment for cardiac failure, it is important to keep in mind that the use of drugs and other therapies aims at improving not only symptoms but also the outcome, or the prognosis, for patients.

Cardiac failure is a chronic disease needing remainder-of-life management. However, with treatment, for many the heart can recover, and the symptoms can improve. Treatment helps the patient live longer and significantly reduces the person's chance of dying suddenly. Sometimes, treating an underlying cause can help. For example, the repair of a heart valve or controlling a fast heart rhythm may ease heart failure symptoms. For most people, treatment involves a balance of the correct medications, lifestyle modifications and, in some cases, surgery and the use of devices that help the heart contract properly.

The two most crucial components to classify cardiac failure are **time** and **function.** The time component relates to whether the heart failure has developed quickly (acute) or slowly (chronic) while the function component is based on the ejection fraction, reduced or preserved.

time

Acute means that cardiac failure comes on rapidly. The person is usually in good health and then presents both unwell and unstable. A hospital emergency department is generally the best place to deal with this situation. The most common conditions that cause acute failure are:

- **coronary artery disease,**
  - **lack of blood flow**, either
    - **complete**, causing a heart attack that paralyses then kills the heart muscle, thus changing the function of the heart, and altering the way it pumps, which can lead to CF or

- **severe lack**, which doesn't necessarily cause the death of the heart muscle, but results in stiffness and failure of the function of the muscle. This changes the pump's action and, so, causes deterioration;

- **heart rhythm change,** where suddenly the heart is beating too quickly or too slowly. This can markedly alter the pump action;

- **infections** that affect the heart, the valves of the heart or the muscle of the heart (as well as infections in other parts of the body) can overdrive the circulation and overload the heart, and

- sudden **valve failure,** where the valve, which should keep the blood flowing in a single direction, allows blood to flow in the opposite direction, thus diminishing the forward flow and the effectiveness of the pump. It can also lead to back-flow and congestion, more often than not, within the lungs.

Chronic cardiac failure presents typically in the clinic. It is usually related to a progressive decompensation of heart-related function, which is secondary to some of the etiologies, or causes, already discussed. These include a lack of blood flow, valves, long-term high blood pressure. It is the day-to-day, week-to-week, people-living-with-it-for-the-rest-of-their-lives scenario.

function

The other way of classifying cardiac failure is in terms of how well the left ventricle is pumping, the ejection fraction. *(refer particularly to pages 35-39)*

commonality

Independent of whether cardiac failure is classified by time or function, an accumulation of fluid in the body – particularly in the lungs – is typical in all cardiac failures. **Diuretic** therapy is the treatment that removes this fluid from the body, by helping the person to pass urine (diuresis).

Diuretic therapy is essential. One specific trigger that leads to cardiac failure is that the body's receptors, in assessing the body's fluid balance, perceive that there is not enough blood flowing around the body. Tricked into thinking that the body has lost blood, the receptors respond by retaining or reabsorbing fluid to re-establish the blood volume back to its 'normal' level. The body then ends up with a very dangerous fluid overload. Under some circumstances, such as blood loss, this receptor system works very well. It doesn't if it is your heart not pumping correctly that initiates the message – in this case, a mis-message – to the body's receptors.

Fluid retention is the consequence of those receptors responding to a sense of diminished blood volume. As mentioned previously, this can manifest itself in swelling of the ankles or legs, or if the fluid collects in the lungs, shortness of breath (and cough). Diuretic therapy clears that fluid and improves people's symptoms. However, an intricate balance is needed. Too much fluid ('wet') and the patient suffers the symptoms; too little fluid ('dry') can stop the kidneys working, as they need fluid passing through them to keep them plump and working well.

Let's say a patient is too 'wet'. I'll ask the patient to take some diuretic therapy for several days in a row, say three, or for three days in a week. This amount of treatment should move the person from being 'wet' to 'dry' but not too 'dry' to risk problems with the kidneys. We then wait to see how long it takes for the fluid to re-accumulate. This time is variable; consumption of fluid, amount and intensity of exercise, and weather are among some of the determining factors. However, the person knows when the symptoms return and goes back on the therapy. I have many patients who move between a little bit 'wet' and a little bit 'dry', responding to their personal needs on a day-to-day basis. It is an excellent help if patients can understand the concept and become involved in their management.

complexities

As cardiac failure is a complex condition with many variants, so is the treatment. Here, we take an overview of treatments available and then, in subsequent chapters, look at them in more detail, in particular, the drug therapies that are available.

drugs

diuretic therapies increase the production of urine and so reduce the amount of fluid in the body, relieving congestion and reducing the strain on the heart. Furosemide (Lasix) is most commonly used.

therapies that block the renin-angiotensin-aldosterone system

The renin-angiotensin-aldosterone system (RAAS) protects the kidneys. It produces aldosterone which keeps sodium in the kidneys, thereby reabsorbing water and increasing fluid volume within the body. Turning off the RAAS releases sodium and water, which then passes out of the body as urine. RAAS blocking therapies include:

- angiotensin-converting enzyme (ACE) inhibitors
- angiotensin II (AT2) receptor blockers
- aldosterone blockers

beta-blockers help dampen the over-drive effect of the sympathetic nervous system (SNS)

neprilysin inhibitors help stop the breakdown of the natriuretic peptides (the good guys)

ivabradine works at the sinus node of the right atrium to slow down the heart rate

digoxin improves the contractility of the heart muscle

hydralazine is a direct smooth muscle relaxant that reduces blood pressure

nitrates are direct smooth muscle relaxants that work on the venous system to reduce the blood flow back to the heart and so 'off-load' the heart

sodium-glucose transport inhibitors

- gliflozins allow salt and sugar to be lost through the urine.

resynchronization therapy re-establishes synchronicity by using a special pacemaker that can overcome the time delay of a bundle branch block

an implantable cardiac defibrillator delivers a shock to the heart to re-establish normal rhythm if the heart develops a potentially fatal rhythm

pulmonary artery blood pressure monitoring

cardiac contractility modulation alters the way calcium in the cells of the heart is utilized, increasing the effectiveness of the muscle contraction

left atrium decompression for people who have heart failure with preserved ejection fraction (under investigation)

blood flow restoration

- stents
- bypass grafting

valve repair or replacement

heart transplant

ventricular assist device, generally an external device that works in conjunction with the patient's own heart, used in the end stages of heart failure to keep the person alive.

non-medical

lifestyle

fluid control

salt intake

regular exercise

yoga and ti-chi

nutritional supplements, including fish oil, co-enzyme Q10 and selenium

diet.

- Cardiac failure is a chronic disease that requires lifelong management.
- With the appropriate care and treatment program
  - symptoms can improve
  - the heart can become stronger
  - the patient can live longer
  - the risk of a person dying suddenly can be reduced.
- Treating any underlying cause/s can help significantly.
- Drug therapies include
  - diuretics
  - ACE inhibitors
  - angiotensin II receptor blockers
  - aldosterone antagonists
  - beta-blockers
  - inotropes (agents that make the heart pump harder)
  - digoxin.
- Non-drug therapies include
  - implanted devices
  - surgical procedures
  - lifestyle changes (dealt with in the next section of the book).

Now, let's look at the drug therapies for cardiac failure more closely. Firstly, diuretics.

Chapter 10
DRUGS – DIURETICS

Diuretics, or 'water pills', are medications that help remove fluid from the body by making the person pass more urine than usual. Potentially, all patients who have symptomatic cardiac failure can use them.

Two types of diuretic drugs interest us, and they are distinguished by where they work in the kidney-urinary system.

Our kidneys and the associated urinary system are quite amazing. Together they receive more than a liter of blood each minute and eliminate about 1.5 liters of urine each day, efficiently ridding the body of excess water and waste products that would otherwise cause serious problems.

As blood flows into the kidney, it goes into the **glomerulus**, the kidney filtration system that filters fluid from the blood. This filtered fluid passes into **collecting tubules** which form into a collecting duct that drains into the bladder through the ureter. The collecting tubules – proximal tubules (near the glomerulus) and distal tubules (further away from the glomerulus) – have different ways of dealing with electrolytes and fluid.

Between the proximal and distal tubules is the **Loop of Henle**. This region is where a further concentration of the urine may occur.

The diuretic drugs we are discussing act at **either** the distal tubule or the Loop of Henle.

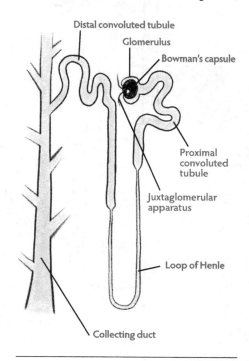

Distal convoluted tubule

Glomerulus

Bowman's capsule

Proximal convoluted tubule

Juxtaglomerular apparatus

Loop of Henle

Collecting duct

kidney detail

Blood flows into each kidney through the **renal artery.** This large blood vessel branches into smaller and smaller blood vessels until the blood reaches the **nephrons.** Each kidney is made up of about 1 million nephrons and each nephron includes a microscopic filter - the **glomerulus,** a cluster of tiny blood vessels - and a tubule. Blood enters the glomerulus by the **afferent** arterioles

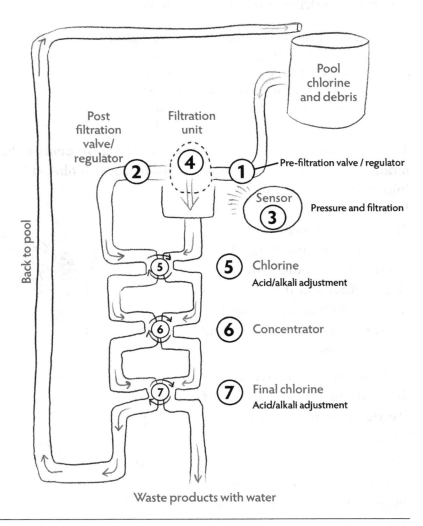

scheme: pool analogy

and leaves by **efferent** arterioles. A blood vessel runs alongside the tubules. Large molecules (such as proteins) and blood cells, stay in the blood vessel while small molecules, wastes and fluid – mostly water – pass through the thin walls of the glomerulus into the tubule. The blood vessel then reabsorbs most of the water, along with minerals and nutrients needed by the body. The waste left in the tubule becomes **urine**. The blood returns to the body via the **renal vein.** The urine passes from the kidneys via the ureters to the bladder.

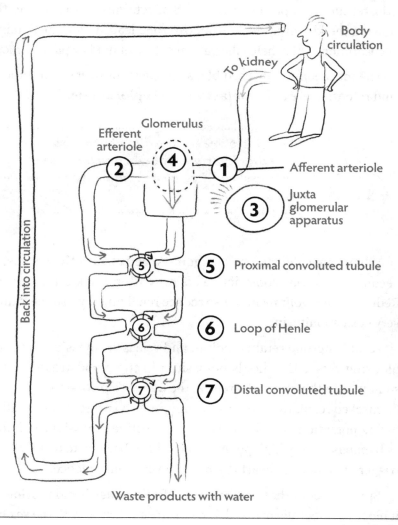

Body circulation

To kidney

Glomerulus

Efferent arteriole

Back into circulation

Afferent arteriole

Juxta glomerular apparatus

(5) Proximal convoluted tubule

(6) Loop of Henle

(7) Distal convoluted tubule

Waste products with water

scheme: body

distal tubule & aldosterone

Mineralocorticoids (*corticoids*, steroid-based hormones; *mineralo*, mineral balance) are hormone messengers that influence electrolyte and water balance in the body. The primary mineralocorticoid is **aldosterone** which acts at the **distal tubule**. There it works to **retain sodium** and therefore, **retain water** and **keep up the fluid level**. Aldosterone blocking agents, or **aldosterone antagonists, are drugs that decrease, and prevent, fluid overload in patients.** They work by blocking aldosterone from performing its job of retaining sodium (and therefore fluid) in the kidneys. Blocking aldosterone leads to a reduction in sodium re-absorption, which helps the patient get rid of fluid by passing more water.

The most commonly used blocking agents or drugs that directly target fluid retention are **spironolactone** and **eplerenone**.

Electrolytes are electrically-charged salts found in the blood that hydrate the body and balance blood acidity and pressure. They also regulate nerve and muscle function.

When using aldosterone antagonists, **renal function** is likely to alter because some vasoconstrictive effects within the kidneys are changed. Reducing fluid volume may also reduce renal function, so the kidneys need very close monitoring.

As aldosterone retains sodium and releases potassium into the urine, blocking this action holds potassium in the bloodstream and releases sodium into the urine. Therefore, the patient's **potassium** level needs to be checked regularly, and the doctor must also ensure that the patient is not taking potassium supplements nor over-eating potassium-rich food, such as bananas. A very high potassium level can become toxic to the heart and trigger an abnormal heart rhythm, a severe consequence.

Spironolactone has another side-effect that needs monitoring. Because it blocks a mineralocorticoid, it has a cross-reaction with the sex hormone,

testosterone, which is produced within the adrenal gland like aldosterone and this can lead to a feminizing effect. For **women,** it could clear up acne or reduce facial hair (not all bad), but for **men,** it could cause uncomfortable breast enlargement (gynecomastia). Swapping spironolactone to eplerenone for men easily fixes the problem. Eplerenone is a newer agent that is more specific than spironolactone. Although, potentially, it has fewer side-effects, it is more expensive than spironolactone.

As with most medications for heart failure, the aldosterone antagonists, in particular spironolactone and eplerenone, are given at a low dose initially and up-titrated over time so as not to affect the patient's hemodynamic (blood flow) balance. Bloods would be checked weekly for the first couple of weeks, then every second or third week, then every fourth week, and then extended, depending on the stability of the patient.

Aldosterone antagonists (blockers) are beneficial with respect to both mortality and morbidity for people with heart failure who have a **reduced ejection fraction** (HFrEF, when the left ventricle is not pumping as well as a healthy heart).

In adding spices to a casserole, you add a little at first and then test the taste, and then add a little bit more, and taste and you keep adding a little more until you achieve the correct flavor. You don't want to overdo it in the first run.

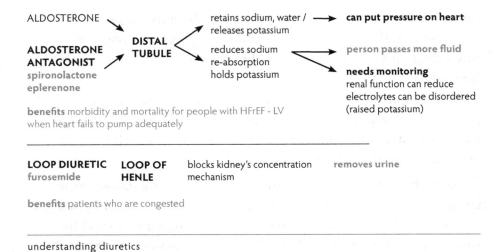

ALDOSTERONE → **DISTAL TUBULE**

ALDOSTERONE ANTAGONIST
spironolactone
eplerenone

retains sodium, water / releases potassium → **can put pressure on heart**

reduces sodium re-absorption
holds potassium → person passes more fluid

→ **needs monitoring**
renal function can reduce
electrolytes can be disordered
(raised potassium)

benefits morbidity and mortality for people with HFrEF - LV when heart fails to pump adequately

---

LOOP DIURETIC   **LOOP OF**   blocks kidney's concentration   removes urine
furosemide   **HENLE**   mechanism

benefits patients who are congested

---

understanding diuretics

Loop of Henle and fluid balance

'Loop' diuretics work by blocking the concentrating mechanisms within the loop of the renal tubule, known as the Loop of Henle.

Fluid balance evaluation is by clinical assessment:

- is the patient short of breath?

- are the person's ankles swollen?

- the jugular venous pulse is checked. The jugular vein connects directly to the right atrium through the superior vena cava, so if there is fluid in the jugular vein, there is high pressure in the right atrium;

- weight, and

- bloods.

The most commonly used agent, **furosemide, blocks the ability of the kidney to concentrate urine.** It is a potent agent for removing large quantities of urine from the body and is particularly useful for significantly congested patients.

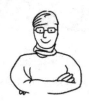

A mineralocorticoid blocker, when used as a diuretic, is often prescribed in conjunction with a loop diuretic. This can augment diuresis as reabsorption of water is blocked in two locations. The doctor then needs to be very careful about fluid balance and fluid loss. Regular blood testing and clinical assessment are essential to ensure the patient is not in fluid over-load or under-load.

The dosage needs to match the response. So, while treatment might start with a low dose to determine how the patient responds, the on-going dosage is based on urine production. However, if a patient presents in a very congested state (fluid overload), a relatively high dose is used initially until the body's water load reduces. Once the patient is close to a good fluid balance, the amount of diuretic therapy is reduced so that the patient does not become too 'dry'. This is important, as long-term dehydration turns off the kidneys. **Not good!**

Is the person drying out too much, or is the balance 'just right'? I encourage patients to use their fluid tablets based on their observations of becoming

- 'too wet', which presents as shortness of breath, swollen ankles and weight gain, or
- 'too dry', which presents as light-headedness from too little fluid in the circulation, thirst, dry skin and dark urine from an increased concentration of fluid.

With those triggers, I ask them to increase or decrease their diuretic therapy slightly to adjust the fluid volume and bring them back to the level we want.

IMPORTANT POINTS

- Diuretic drugs remove fluid from the body by making the person pass more urine.
- They can be used for all patients who have symptomatic cardiac failure.
- There are two types of drugs prescribed, depending on where they work
    - distal tubule (aldosterone antagonists – spironolactone and eplerenone)
    - Loop of Henle (loop diuretic – furosemide).
- Care needs to be taken with fluid balance when the two types of drugs are used together.

drugs — ACE inhibitors

chapter 11
DRUGS – ACE INHIBITORS

ACE inhibitors are medications indicated for patients whose hearts are not pumping well, that is, for hearts with **reduced** ejection fraction (HFrEF).

After several landmark trials, **angiotensin-converting enzyme (ACE) inhibitors** came into widespread use during the 1990s as powerful agents in the treatment and management of congestive heart failure in individuals with **decreased left ventricle function**, or **reduced contraction** of the heart. The first agent that really set the stage was **captopril**. Significant data showed outcomes of improved quality of life and, more significantly, improved morbidity and mortality. Since then, several other similar drugs, including **enalapril**, **perindopril** and **ramipril**, have been developed. The less frequent dosing with these newer agents is comfortable and convenient for patients to take and also easier to remember, so less likely to be missed. The newer agents have equal efficacy to captopril.

The angiotensin-converting enzyme (ACE) is the enzyme that converts angiotensin I (AT1) to angiotensin II (AT2). **AT2** works on the angiotensin II receptor, and causes vasoconstriction, which **keeps up blood pressure**. As AT2 **constricts** the small efferent arteriole that leaves the glomerulus, it **increases filtration**. The production of aldosterone, the hormone that acts at the kidney to absorb sodium, is also stimulated, ensuring that water stays within the circulation, maintaining blood volume.

Such a response is very sensible if you are bleeding profusely from a cut on the leg out on the African Plains two million years ago. You would want to maintain your blood pressure and your renal function and have a plan to reabsorb more fluid to re-establish your body's fluid balance. Unfortunately, the action of the AT2 receptor is detrimental if your heart is not working properly. So, by taking an **ACE inhibitor** tablet and **preventing the conversion of AT1 to AT2,** the function of the AT2 receptor is down-regulated, thus mitigating those effects that can be counter-productive for the failing heart.

side-effects

As we introduce these drugs, however, the very things we want them to do can give rise to **side-effects**: blood pressure, kidney function, aldosterone levels and cough. These side-effects need on-going monitoring.

If you think about it, this makes perfect sense. If we're giving someone an agent that is turning off a vasoconstrictor (that helps maintain renal function and a pathway that maintains sodium at the expense of potassium), guess what the side-effects might be? Correct! Lower blood pressure, reduced renal function and raised potassium levels.

blood pressure

If we give patients an ACE inhibitor, we can lower their blood pressure and make them hypotensive (*hypo*, low; *tensive*, blood pressure). Although the pressure needs to be low, it does not need to be so low that each time the person stands up he or she feels like falling over. So, the introduction of these agents needs to be careful and gradual, while keeping a close watch on the blood pressure.

kidney function

If we give patients an ACE inhibitor, it lessens the constriction on the efferent arteriole leaving the glomerulus, and so reduces the amount of flow going through the filtration unit. This needs a gentle approach, otherwise, it can lead to a significant reduction in renal function, and that is **a problem**. As the ACE inhibitor is added to the therapeutic regime, the glomerular filtration rate, which measures the filtration that impacts the kidney function, needs to be maintained as well as possible. Increasing the amount of ACE inhibitor slowly, over time as the body adjusts, helps to reduce potential renal problems.

aldosterone levels

As aldosterone maintains sodium at the expense of potassium, any reduction in aldosterone action via ACE inhibitors can lead to increased potassium levels in the blood. Increased potassium levels can lead to significant side-effects:

- nervousness
- confusion
- irregular heartbeat
- shortness of breath
- difficulty with breathing
- tingling or numbness in hands, feet or lips
- weakness or a feeling a heaviness in the legs.

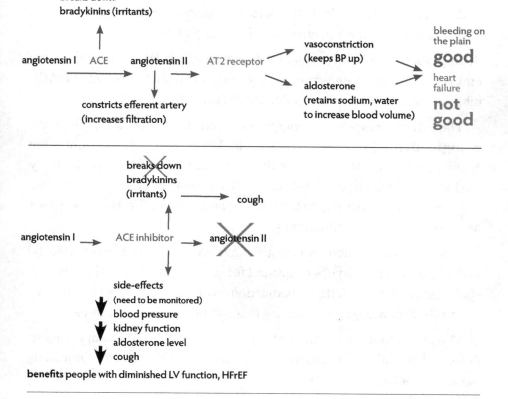

It is very important, therefore, that renal function and sodium and potassium levels are regularly checked (initially, weekly) through blood tests.

cough

As well as breaking down AT1 to AT2, the angiotensin-converting enzyme (ACE) also breaks down **bradykinins** to inactive products. Bradykinins are part of the calcarine system. Although they are not well understood, they have a role in inflammation, vasodilation and cell migration. They also have a role in pain, and so it is thought that they are involved with tissue injury. Bradykinins seem to have irritant properties of their own, and the ACE breaks these down into inactive components. Use of an ACE inhibitor, therefore, can lead to a reduction in the breakdown of these potentially irritant compounds such that, in a few people, this can produce its own symptoms. The most common symptom is a cough. So, ACE inhibition leading to reduced bradykinin breakdown can irritate the lining of the lungs, resulting in a dry, unproductive cough for the patient.

Importantly, as a cough can be a symptom of cardiac failure, the doctor and patient need to determine if the cough is a side-effect of the ACE inhibitor **or** an indication of under-treatment of CF.

The extreme response of cough in the setting of bradykinin elevation is **angioedema** (*angio*, blood vessel; *oedema*, swelling). Not only is the cough present but there is also swelling around the face, and particularly the tongue that could block the airway. This severe allergic-type response requires an immediate trip to the hospital and dictates that the person **not** be exposed to an ACE inhibitor again.

I use these ACE inhibitors as first-line agents partly because they were the first available. They have been around for several decades, so there is long clinical experience with these medications with excellent patient outcomes and well-acknowledged side-effects that can be carefully monitored.

The aim is to increase these ACE inhibitors to the maximum tolerated dose, without side-effects, as maximum blockage of the AT2 receptor leads to the best outcome for the CF patient.

There is a happy ending to the story even if there is a small reduction in renal function when these drugs are first introduced. In the long term, ACE inhibitors are renal-protective. They look after the kidneys over years and decades.

IMPORTANT POINTS

- There is a tension in cardiac failure between
  - the **heart**, which needs low blood pressure and less fluid volume to pump, and
  - the **kidneys,** which need fluid volume and good blood pressure to work correctly.
- ACE inhibitors are for patients with HFrEF.
- The angiotensin-converting enzyme (ACE) converts angiotensin I (AT1) to angiotensin II (AT2) which works on the AT2 receptor. This is not good for a heart in cardiac failure as it creates a fluid overload and places strain on the heart that could be detrimental.
- The ACE inhibitor drugs down-regulate the AT2 receptor.
- Side-effects – problems with blood pressure, kidney function, aldosterone levels, cough – need to be monitored closely.
- Renal failure and cardiac failure are not happy bed fellows and one cannot be favored at the expense of the other
  - renal function must be monitored closely
  - potassium levels must be monitored closely.
- Is a cough an ACE inhibitor side-effect or under-treated CF?

drugs — the angiotensin II (AT2) receptor blockers

chapter 12
DRUGS – AT2 RECEPTOR BLOCKERS

Remember the renin-angiotensin-aldosterone system (RAAS) and the responses that the body puts in place to constrict the efferent arteriole leaving the filtering unit of the kidney, the glomerulus? Recall, too, the mechanisms used to raise the hormone, aldosterone, to hold sodium, and therefore water, in the bloodstream and so increase blood volume? The AT2 receptor drives much of that action.

Signals from changes in blood pressure affect the juxtaglomerular cells near the glomerulus and the hormone, renin, is released. Via a series of enzymatic processes through the body, renin leads to the formation of AT2, which has the role of vascular constriction of the blood vessel that leaves the glomerulus, the efferent arteriole. This ensures that the kidneys continue to produce urine despite low blood pressure. The AT2 receptor also drives the production of aldosterone, which works at the kidneys to keep sodium and water in the bloodstream. If your heart is not working well, these normal physiological responses can be detrimental.

AT2 receptor blockers (ARB) act directly on the AT2 receptor in the RAAS. ACE inhibitors work on the same system. However, they work higher up the pathway where they prevent the conversion of AT1 to AT2. The AT2 blocker agents work at the receptor on the final step of that same pathway. As expected, both drugs produce very similar results.

These AT2 receptor blocker agents, primarily those commonly used in clinical practice such as **candesartan** and **valsartan**, can be used for blood pressure as well, and, just like the ACE inhibitors, improve outcomes for patients who have diminished left ventricular function, HFrEF. The AT2 receptor blockers:

- lower blood pressure by blocking vasoconstriction, so they help the body's blood vessels relax and dilate

- diminish filtration through the kidney by relaxing the efferent arteriole, and

- lessen the production of aldosterone.

AT2 blockers are administered in the same way as ACE inhibitors; the dosage is started low and gradually increased.

The side-effects are very similar. However, because AT2 blockers do not interfere with the bradykinin system, as do the ACE inhibitors, cough and angioedema are rare side-effects.

As these drugs are being up-titrated, regular blood tests are needed to ensure that the kidney function does not drop off too much and that the potassium levels do not go too high.

The most important thing is that your doctor closely monitors your renal function when using these agents, at least for the first few weeks, and then lengthening the time between tests.

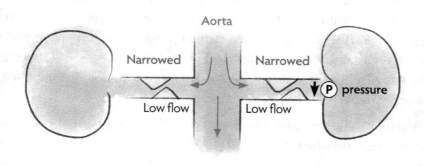

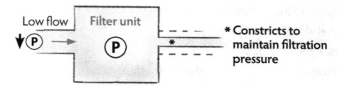

Dilation in filtration unit

caused by ACE or AT2 blocker

In very rare circumstances, the kidney function can drop dramatically if there is a significant impairment to blood flow to the two kidneys, simultaneously. A narrowing of both renal arteries, called **bilateral renal artery stenosis**, RAS, can cause this. Both ACE inhibitors and AT2 blockers can precipitate this marked reduction in renal function. That is because the low flow to the kidneys (caused by a narrowed renal artery) is compensated for by a tight or restricted blood vessel leaving the glomerulus, so maintaining filtration. However, this is the very blood vessel on which the ACE inhibitor and AT2 blockers act.

In my experience, patients new to using these agents may experience low blood pressure as the main side-effect, describing light-headedness on rising from a sitting or lying position, particularly if the movement is after some time of stillness. Often, I invite patients to take these blood pressure agents at night. Some data suggest benefit from taking the medication in the evening, and as the majority of heart-related events occur in the 'wee hours' of the morning, night-time dosing seems sensible for symptoms and prognosis. Furthermore, from a practical perspective, if taken at night, there is a reasonable chance that the lower blood pressure effect occurs while lying in bed and, so, the person is not as aware of the change in pressure, compared to during times of activity during the day.

Generally, **AT2 receptor blockers should not be given at the same time as ACE inhibitors, although they are interchangeable**. As agents, they are too similar and if used together could dampen the RAAS too much, causing other, unwanted, problems. ACE inhibitors are my preferred first-line agents as they have been in use for the longer time and have the most data to support them. However, there are patients who, for various reasons, do not tolerate ACE inhibitors. For example, a patient who has an irritating cough, or has suffered angioedema after taking an ACE inhibitor, is an ideal candidate for the use of an AT2 receptor blocker.

Increasing numbers of preparations are coming on to the market that combine two, or even three, different classes of drugs in a single tablet for the convenience of the patient.

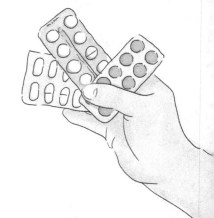

Perhaps if you are on a 'handful' of tablets, ask your doctor if any come in a 'combo' to reduce the number of tablets you need to take.

NSAIDs

Renal failure and cardiac failure are not happy bedfellows. Care must be taken around not only fluid balance but other factors, including drugs, that could impact kidney function. Necessary, front-of-mind considerations include the use of **non-steroidal anti-inflammatory drugs** (NSAID) such as Nurofen and Voltaren. Such drugs are fantastic for helping people with arthritis move. Since many cardiac failure sufferers are older members of the community, they may well benefit from the use of NSAIDs if they have a few aches and pains. The problem is that these drugs can have detrimental effects on the kidneys, and, in some cases, not just worsen renal function but **precipitate renal failure**.

NSAIDs reduce the production of chemical messengers called prostaglandins. **Prostaglandins** are responsible for inflammatory responses, and part of that includes relaxing or dilating blood vessels. The redness and heat of inflammation are from the increase in blood flow. There are local prostaglandins in the kidney that specifically act on the artery that **enters** the glomerulus, the **afferent** arteriole. NSAIDs reduce renal prostaglandins and so the afferent arteriole constricts, resulting in less pressure and less blood flow into the glomerulus. If also using an ACE inhibitor or AT2 blocker — both leading to relaxation of the artery that **leaves** the glomerulus, the **efferent** arteriole — then possible filtration has been reduced from 'both ends' of the process. This can be a **disaster**.

As prostaglandins also protect the lining of the stomach, aspirin and NSAIDs are linked to ulcers. They also cause uterine contraction during menstruation, hence NSAIDs are beneficial for period pain.

My practice is to follow the guidelines and use mineralocorticoid blockers regularly for my patients with reduced ejection cardiac failure (HFrEF). I also prescribe the loop diuretic, furosemide, on an as-needed basis. I ask that when the body collects some fluid, the patient takes the furosemide tablet for a few days, loses that fluid, stops the furosemide and waits until the fluid re-accumulates before retaking the medication. This timing gives the kidneys a chance to recover.

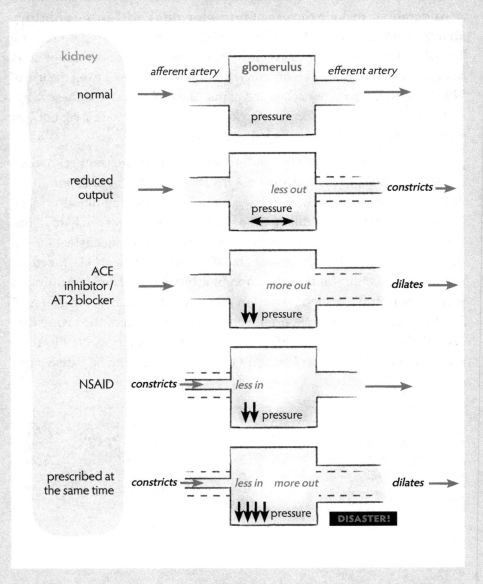

Just think about it. While we're drying a patient out using a distal tubular diuretic and a loop diuretic and then add in a non-steroidal anti-inflammatory drug, we've just created a heady cocktail to turn off that patient's kidneys. And that spells disaster!

Then, concerning the NSAIDs, I explain that I would love my patients to be pain-free every day; I would love them to be able to take these tablets all the time. However, it is just not safe.

My suggestion is to use the non-steroidal anti-inflammatory drugs two, or maybe three, days a week at the most to give the kidneys a chance to recover. I suggest they take them on the day they play bowls, the day they go shopping, the day the grandkids come around; in other words, take them on their more active days of the week. The days they have a rest, their kidneys can have a rest, too. As an alternative to NSAIDs, I remind patients that taking their paracetamol regularly works well, much better than 'as needed', and is safe at recommended doses.

Although it is really important to help people be free of the symptoms of cardiac failure, it is also essential that the body is not damaged further by shutting down the kidneys or pushing the potassium to unacceptably high, or even dangerous, levels.

While there are no good current studies that demonstrate that treating the fluid with loop diuretics improves outcome, it certainly makes patients feel better. Optimistically, some data suggest, however, that treating the fluid balance really carefully will make a prognostic difference. There are trials currently underway (early 2021) looking at this.

Angiotensin II receptor blockers are

- great medications to
  - lower blood pressure
  - decrease filtration through the kidneys
  - alter aldosterone production, thereby reducing sodium retention so that sodium is lost, and potassium retained
- 10 years 'younger' than ACE inhibitors
- similar, but not the same as ACE inhibitors; they work on different parts of the same pathway
- can be used interchangeably with ACE inhibitors but not used at the same time
- the go-to medication for the patient who does not tolerate ACE inhibitors

Non-steroidal anti-inflammatory drugs (NSAIDs) should be used sparingly.

drugs — beta-blockers

chapter 13
DRUGS – BETA-BLOCKERS

What is 'beta' and what is blocked?

As previously mentioned, the body's nervous system, the autonomic nervous system, has two components, the sympathetic nervous system (SNS) and the parasympathetic nervous system (PSNS).

The **sympathetic nervous system** is like an **accelerator** that powers up the nervous system into a 'fight or flight' response. This response gets you going if someone or something threatens you; if you're scared. Your heart rate increases, the blood goes to your legs, your pupils dilate. Everything within your body is ready to fight or run.

On the other hand, the **parasympathetic nervous system** is like a **brake** that slows down the body. It is the one that says, "Let's slow down and digest what we've just eaten", the 'rest and digest' response. This response moves the body into downtime when the body is recuperating, such as when sleeping or digesting.

Our interest here is the **sympathetic nervous system** (SNS). When the heart is in cardiac failure, the body receives signals that the heart is not doing its job properly. The SNS kicks in to **compensate** for the decrease in cardiac output. The SNS operates through alpha and beta receptors. Beta receptors, therefore, are part of the receptor system that up-regulates the body's response to a problem. They are the target for beta blockade. Beta-blockers, as used in treating cardiac failure, target the beta receptor pathway and **dampen the over-drive effect of the SNS**. A high density of beta receptors in the heart is the target of this therapy. More specifically, a subgroup, **beta2 receptors**, is targeted as there are also beta1 receptors that help dilate the airways, and we don't want to interfere with that.

When these agents first came into use, doctors were very cautious about using beta blockade in cardiac failure. If you're dealing with a patient who already has a poorly functioning heart, to give medication that might

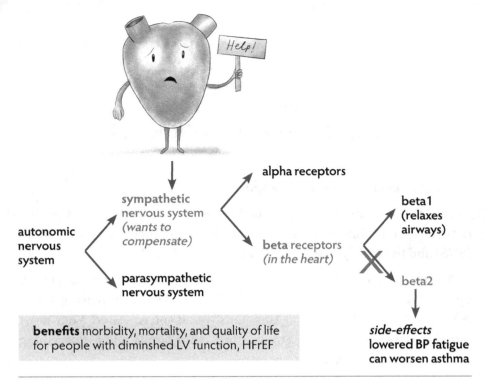

benefits morbidity, mortality, and quality of life for people with diminshed LV function, HFrEF

side-effects lowered BP fatigue can worsen asthma

autonomic nervous system

dampen that function even further is a scary thought. As it happens, by initially using a 'trickle' of beta-blocker and gradually increasing it (to avoid blood pressure upset by the drop in cardiac function), a highly beneficial effect is achieved by dampening the sympathetic drive.

Several agents are now available for patients whose left ventricular function is reduced (HFrEF). These agents include **carvedilol, bisoprolol,** an extended-release **metoprolol** preparation, and **nebivolol**. These agents are relatively long-acting and can be gently up-titrated as required. All the research says that their use improves mortality, morbidity and quality of life for people with reduced cardiac function.

These agents are mostly well tolerated. Because they offset the action of the SNS, however, side-effects can be predicted: lowered blood pressure and a feeling of fatigue.

Provided the blood pressure does not become too low, this can be good for the recovery of the heart. As blood pressure is the work that the heart does, day in and day out, at the very least, it would ensure less burden on the heart.

While blood pressure is significant in the setting of cardiac failure, it is crucial not to bring it down too much, nor too quickly. So, the beta-blockers are started at a low dosage and up-titrated, slowly and carefully, with close assessment of how the patient is responding.

The patient's heart rate response also needs to be considered. It is a good sympathetic blockade if the heart rate is under about 70-odd beats a minute, and, generally, no lower than 50 beats a minute at rest.

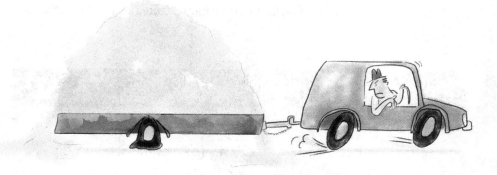

If the head gasket of your car was a bit dodgy, would you drive around in that car pulling a trailer load of sand? The work your heart 'engine' has to do is directly related to the blood pressure 'trailer'.

As the beta blockade is down-regulating one of the drivers of the body, some patients experience fatigue or lethargy. If this becomes a problem, there are several ways to move forward:

- change the prescribed beta-blocker
- change it to a night-time dose to offset some of the day-time effects
- lower the dose or up-titrate more gradually, hoping that the patient becomes accustomed to any ongoing fatigue.

Another issue that can arise is that beta-blockers can affect the airways of the lungs, as the bronchial tubes dilate when the sympathetic drive increases. People living with asthma who are sensitive to any airway constriction can have problems.

That beta-blockers can worsen asthma is really important.

Fortunately, it is not too common. However, for the people in this subset, the clinician needs to decide if the shortness of breath (or even just an irritating cough) in someone who has cardiac failure and asthma is worsening heart function or asthma because of the beta-blocker. If it is

- asthma – then that needs appropriate therapy;
- asthma from the beta-blocker – then beta blockade may not be the appropriate therapy for that individual's heart failure, or
- not asthma – the cardiac failure treatment strategies need reassessing.

IMPORTANT POINTS

Beta-blockers

- target the beta2 receptor pathway (part of the SNS)
- dampen the SNS over-drive effect
- are generally well-tolerated
- are long-lasting and can be gently up-titrated
- improve mortality, morbidity, and quality of life
- have predictable side-effects
  - lowered blood pressure
  - fatigue
  - can worsen asthma

Let's now look at the more specialized medications.

chapter 14
DRUGS – NEXT LINE

The drug therapies already discussed form the starting point for treatment. There are more drug possibilities, including neprilysin inhibitors, ivabradine, digoxin, hydralazine and nitrates, and sodium-glucose transport inhibitors.

neprilysin inhibitors

Neprilysin inhibitors are drugs that **stop** the **breakdown** of the natriuretic peptides. As reducing the breakdown of those favorable peptides keeps their levels higher, the use of neprilysin inhibitors produces positive effects.

The natriuretic peptide system takes stress off the heart when the heart sends out chemical messengers that it is under excessive load. The natriuretic peptides give rise to favorable changes in the circulation to support ongoing heart function. These peptides **decrease**:

- **vasoconstriction**, lowering blood pressure, making it easier for the heart to work;

- **sympathetic tone**, the part of the autonomic nervous system that drives and up-regulates heart rate, and also drives blood pressure. Decreasing sympathetic tone reduces stress and strain on the heart;

- **aldosterone levels**. Aldosterone is the hormone that helps the kidneys to retain sodium so that the body retains fluid. As this can increase blood pressure, blocking aldosterone helps lower blood pressure;

- **inflammation** and **fibrosis** in the heart. This is very important in the long term as an inflamed and fibrotic heart becomes stiff and does not work well;

- the progression of **dysfunctional remodeling** of the left ventricle. If the heart is under stress, it can respond by thickening, and thickened hearts do not work as well as healthy hearts. So, the natriuretic peptides reduce that progression, modifying it favorably;

- the **volume of fluid** in the body by promoting natriuresis, or the passing of fluid. Reducing total fluid volume lessens the work of the circulatory system for the heart.

Despite all their benefits, neprilysin inhibitors can have a **toxic effect on renal function.** Because they alter the way the vascular bed performs, this affects how the blood vessels leaving the glomerulus work. Neprilysin inhibitors can also **lower blood pressure**. They need careful, slow titration so that the patient can cope with the drug.

These agents are beneficial for people with **reduced ejection fraction.** Currently, they are not the first-line agents but are brought into play when the patient is not progressing as well as expected or if the function of the left ventricle remains depressed.

Researchers in a recent trial, Paragon HF[6], tried to assess if these agents could help patients with preserved ejection fraction cardiac failure and the results were not as encouraging as had been hoped. This might be a future area of interest.

The clinically-available neprilysin inhibitor is called **sacubitril**. It is available as a combination medication used in association with an AT2 receptor blocker. The combination means that the renin-angiotensin-aldosterone-axis and the natriuretic peptide axis can be dealt with simultaneously. This combination has a fantastic effect on outcome.

Neprilysin inhibitors cannot be used in conjunction with ACE inhibitors. Some of the breakdown products that are increased with the ACE inhibitors and some of the breakdown products that are increased with the neprilysin inhibitors can interact to significantly increase the likelihood of angioedema developing. Not good!

ivabradine

Sympathetic tone increases the heart rate, driving poorer outcomes. Research suggests that an agent that can bring the heart rate down, used in isolation, could lead to beneficial outcomes for people with **reduced ejection fraction** cardiac failure.

The agent, **ivabradine**, works in the **right atrium** at the **sinus node,** where the heartbeat speed is determined. Ivabradine acts as a blocker to a particular electrolyte channel, **slowing** the repolarization of those cells in the 'pacemaker' center of the heart, and thus, slowing down the heart rate.

Ivabradine tends to be used when a patient's heart rate is over about 75 beats per minute in the resting state. Useful data are showing that if ivabradine does slow the heart rate, an improved outcome for the individual and improved symptomatic control are likely. The drug is generally very well tolerated.

As with other heart failure medications, ivabradine is introduced with a low dosage and gradually increased. The aim is to achieve a heart rate at rest between 50 and 60 beats per minute.

hydralazine and nitrates

Before the advent of the ACE inhibitors, drugs were used that would lead to dilatation of the blood vessels through different mechanisms. Two agents, in particular, are **hydralazine**, which is a direct smooth muscle relaxant, and **nitrates**, also a smooth muscle relaxant that works predominantly on the venous side.

Hydralazine and nitrates, in combination, lead to decreased blood pressure on the arterial side while opening up the vascular bed on the venous side. Although the body can become a little congested by opening up the venous side, the benefit is that it creates diminished 'available' total vascular volume. This, then, 'off-loads' the heart.

Hydralazine and nitrates still work. However, today they are generally kept for people who do not tolerate the ACE inhibitors or the AT2 receptor blockers.

CASE STUDY – MARTIN

young, left bundle branch block,
raised troponin levels, dilated LV, HFrEF,
regional wall motion abnormalities,
dilated cardiomyopathy, bicuspid aortic valve

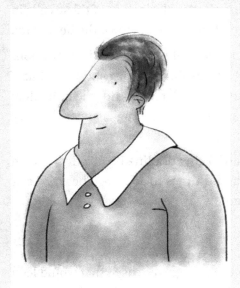

Martin was only in his 30s, married and seemed to be well when he presented to the hospital with nonspecific chest pain.

At the time of his evaluation in accident and emergency, he was found to have a left bundle branch block. This condition shows as an ECG pattern. The electrical trace indicates that the passage of electricity through the main chambers of the heart is slightly disordered. It means that one of the electrical 'wires' that should be distributing the electrical signal to the ventricles is not working. These wires are called Purkinje Fibers. When one malfunctions, the signal is forced to move through the ventricle differently, from cell to cell, rather than through the fibers which, when operating properly, distribute that electrical current evenly throughout the ventricles simultaneously. A blood test showed elevated troponin levels. Troponin is a marker for strain on the heart muscle.

I was asked to see this young man because there was concern that he may have had damage to his heart through a blocked artery. Under most circumstances, this would possibly be the most common cause of his symptoms. However, it is very uncommon in a man this young, and there was no family history of heart problems.

An echocardiogram showed that Martin had

- *a dilated left ventricle, so his heart was bigger than expected;*

- *regional wall motion abnormality due to the dissynchrony caused by the left bundle branch block;*

- *an ejection fraction (EF) of 35-to-40 percent (low), and*

- *as an incidental finding, two leaflets for his aortic valve (a bicuspid aortic valve) rather than the standard three leaflets (tricuspid aortic valve). A bicuspid aortic valve presents its own issues in the longer term. A two-leaflet aortic valve tends to have less balance and, therefore, experiences more wear and tear than a three-leaflet valve, leading to a higher risk of Martin requiring surgery during his lifetime.*

As a bicuspid aortic valve is mostly an inherited condition developing in utero, it is present from birth. It is twice as common in men as it is in women.

As it was important to ascertain the health of Martin's arteries, I organized a CT coronary angiogram, which is a non-invasive way to evaluate the arteries. At this stage, I didn't think I was seeing a typical blocked coronary artery pattern or presentation but, more likely, a dilated cardiomyopathy. I thought that his arteries would be disease-free.

Coronary imaging confirmed my thoughts; his arteries were pristine. There wasn't a blockage, and more importantly, his arteries did not even contain any early plaque.

This was beneficial information as plaque in the arteries could have become a problem in the future.

These findings supported a working diagnosis of dilated cardiomyopathy (dilated, the ventricle is bigger than it should be; cardio, the heart; myo, muscle; pathy, disease). I immediately started Martin on the appropriate therapy for this condition: a beta-blocker, carvedilol, an ACE inhibitor, ramipril, and the diuretic, spironolactone.

Interestingly, Martin had described very little in the way of symptoms. He said he had been lethargic from time to time, but not in terms of limiting function. And he certainly lived a normal life without any reference to impairment or disability or diminished exercise capacity from shortness of breath.

I followed Martin closely over the coming weeks and I up-titrated the beta-blocker and the ACE inhibitor. Measurable improvement was achieved based on measured EF, now over 40 percent. Interestingly, again, Martin reported very little in terms of improvement, although he did describe intermittent fatigue and tiredness. I thought this might have related to the beta blockade, and so I swapped one long-acting beta-blocker for another one. Sometimes the different agents can be tolerated differently by individuals.

Everything seemed to be going very well. With his improvement, I thought there must have been some transient impact on his heart which had been stabilized by the therapies. Hopefully, the heart was now healing itself. With a great deal of optimism, I looked forward to seeing him some 12 months later and booked him in for an ultrasound at that time.

When I saw him, he had experienced – about a month to six weeks before – a mystery illness that had put him in hospital for nearly a week. He had had fevers and was just generally unwell. There was no clear-cut diagnosis. Nobody knew what it was. A mystery. But it did sound like an infective illness. Importantly, though, his repeat echocardiogram showed that his ejection function had slipped back to 35-40 percent. This function had dropped off without a great deal of clinical symptomatology, and not much on examination findings either. However, it was clear, through the echo, that his LV (left ventricular) function had diminished.

With that drop-off in function, I thought it was important to up-regulate his therapy. I took him off the ACE inhibitor and added entresto, a neprilysin inhibitor-AT2 receptor blocker combination. The aim was to increase our impact on the RAAS and the neprilysin system. I wanted to down-regulate the renin-aldosterone system while up-regulating the 'helpful' neprilysin system.

Well, I've kept a close eye on him since. We found that his heart rate, even on maximum therapy, was still on the high side, at over 77 beats a minute at rest. With that being the case, I have added ivabradine to his therapeutic regime. This agent works in the right atrium, at the node that controls the heart rate, to reduce the heartbeat rate.

Interestingly, because of his young age, we have had the chance to check his father's LV function. His father's EF was at 50 percent, which is at the lower end of the normal range. We found, too, that his father does not have a bicuspid aortic valve. Also, we are arranging for Martin to undergo genetic testing to evaluate if there is a clear marker for his dilated cardiomyopathy. This result could be important for his siblings, and certainly, as he's married and hoping to have children in the future, it could be very important for planning pregnancies.

I'm looking forward to seeing Martin at his next visit. I'm hoping that, as the mystery illness recedes, our interventions with maximal therapy will allow his heart to improve. We need to follow that bundle branch block because, if it is severe, devices can improve the distribution of the electrical signal into the heart. This resynchronization therapy is something we may need to consider for Martin in the longer term. Bicuspid aortic valve follow-up (including being aware of this inherited condition for his children) and assessment of possible genetic predisposition for dilated cardiomyopathy are also part of his ongoing journey.

Although Martin did not exhibit much in the way of symptoms, he presents a compelling, ongoing case.

digoxin

Another (surprising) agent successfully being used as an add-on therapy for heart failure is **digoxin**. This drug comes from the foxglove plant and has been used for hundreds of years. Its current-day use is mostly in the management of atrial fibrillation (AF) where it slows down the electrical conduction from the top of the heart to the bottom of the heart. In cardiac failure, it has a small role in improving the **contractility of the myocardium**, the muscle of the heart.

Care is needed when using digoxin. Dosage should be titrated, and results monitored closely. Digoxin is metabolized, or cleared, by the kidneys. So, if diuretic therapy and blood pressure tablets that could impact kidney function are also being used, the digoxin level needs scrutiny. If it goes too high, the patient can become toxic, with the first sign being nausea or not wanting to eat.

However, digoxin assists diminished left ventricular function for people who are in normal sinus rhythm. Patients who are in atrial fibrillation also find it helpful as it regulates their heart rate.

Although some studies using digoxin in people with normal sinus rhythm and heart failure have not shown improvement in mortality, its use reduces hospitalization time, and that's a good outcome for everyone.

sodium-glucose transport inhibitors

In very recent times, one of the most exciting advances for making a difference for people suffering cardiac failure, particularly in people who also have **diabetes**, is with a group of drugs called the **gliflozins** or sodium-glucose transport inhibitors (SGLT2 inhibitors), and, initially, one in particular, **empagliflozin**, as others are coming through. The EMPA-REG OUTCOME trial[7], a diabetes trial, demonstrated, surprisingly to the investigators, that there was a significant reduction in cardiac failure in the active treatment group.

Gliflozin agents (including empagliflozin) are drugs that work at the **proximal tubule** of the kidney, **shutting down sodium-glucose transport.** This means that sodium and glucose that have been filtered by the glomerulus are not reabsorbed in the proximal tubule as is generally the case, allowing the loss of salt and sugar into the urine. Remember, retained salt leads to retained fluid which leads to elevated blood pressure. **Not good.**

Using these agents has shown a clear benefit in the reduction of mortality and reduction of hospitalizations with improved quality of life for diabetic patients with cardiac failure.

Losing some sodium is good. Losing sugar takes water with it as well.

The gliflozins are under extensive investigation. The release of the DAPA HF trial[8] at the European Society of Cardiology meeting in Paris in 2019 showed the SGLT2 inhibitor **dapagliflozin** was a beneficial add-on therapy for cardiac failure patients already appropriately treated regardless of whether or not they had diabetes.

Amazingly, a class of drugs that started 'life' as a treatment for diabetes is about to become a central pillar of cardiac failure treatment. There's no question that exciting times are ahead with these new agents becoming more available for clinical use.

IMPORTANT POINTS

Further drug treatment possibilities for cardiac failure include **neprilysin inhibitors**

- stop the breakdown of the natriuretic peptides,
- can have a toxic effect on the renal system,
- often used in combination with AT2 receptor blockers,
- cannot be used with ACE inhibitors

(continued next page)

ivabradine

- works in the right atrium to slow the heart rate
- is well tolerated

hydralazine and nitrates

- older drugs that are now used for people who do not tolerate ACE inhibitors and AT2 receptor blockers

digoxin

- more commonly used in AF treatment,
- in the CF setting, it can improve the myocardium's contractility

sodium-glucose transport inhibitors

- new drugs that have come to CF attention through treatment for diabetes

[6]   Prospective Comparison of ARNI With ARB Global Outcomes in HF With Preserved Ejection Fraction - PARAGON-HF. American College of Cardiology; date presented. 30 March 2020; date published 26 April 2021.
https://www.acc.org/latest-in-cardiology/clinical-trials/2019/08/30/21/24/paragon-hf

[7]   Empagliflozin, Cardiovascular Outcomes, and Mortality in Type 2 Diabetes or EMPA-REG trial. The New England Journal of Medicine November 26 2015
https://www.nejm.org/doi/full/10.1056/nejmoa1504720

[8]   Dapagliflozin in Patients with Heart Failure and Reduced Ejection Fraction or DAPA-HF trial. The New England Journal of Medicine November 21 20219
https://www.nejm.org/doi/full/10.1056/NEJMoa1911303

We will now look at the various devices and procedures currently used to treat cardiac failure.

chapter 15
IMPLANTED DEVICES AND SURGICAL PROCEDURES

Help for patients in cardiac failure extends beyond medications to devices and procedures.

saving a life

Patients with cardiac failure can suffer cardiac arrest and, literally, drop dead. If a person

- survives cardiac arrest, **or**
- survives sustained lethal rhythms of the heart such as ventricular tachycardia, **and**
- has a reduced ejection fraction of less than 40 percent,

then the research suggests that consideration should be given to **implanting a device** to save that person's life in the future should such an event occur again.

That device is an **implantable cardiac defibrillator**. It is a small battery-powered device with wires that go into the heart. This implantable cardiac defibrillator does the same job as do the paddles that are used on the chest during cardiac arrest when hearts are 'shocked' (as you have no doubt seen during television programs and in the movies), except from the inside!

The patient then has a device that is constantly monitoring the heart and is 'ready for action' 24 hours a day, seven days a week, until the battery needs changing, which is about five to eight years. If there is a problem and the patient 'dies', the implantable cardiac defibrillator kicks the heart back to life. It is a fantastic technology that is highly recommended if an individual with a bad heart suffers such an event. Here, it is **secondary** prevention as it **prevents** a second cardiac event.

To reduce heart muscle damage from a heart attack, people ideally need to be treated within 90 minutes of their first symptom. Such treatment includes clot-busting or inserting a stent to open the artery.

There are situations, however, where cardiologists implant these devices as **primary** prevention **before** a person has had a serious event, wanting to **prevent** the first event. These are generally patients who have had a heart attack and suffered significant impairment to the function of their left ventricle, through lack of blood supply. Such an occurrence is called **ischemic** heart disease (*ischemic,* lack of blood flow).

It takes until about six weeks after the heart attack before an assessment of the left ventricular function can be made, as the ventricle needs time to

AN IMPLANTABLE CARDIAC DEFIBRILLATOR
(does not equal) A PACEMAKER

*An implantable cardiac defibrillator is similar to a permanent pacemaker in its appearance and implantation but is very different in its function. The **pacemaker** provides tiny electrical impulses to trigger the heart, similar to the body's own electrical signal. The **defibrillator** discharges a much larger electrical impulse, so large it is called a 'shock' and used when the heart is in a life-threatening rhythm. The shock stops the life-threatening rhythm and lets the heart 'restart'.*

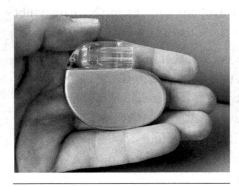

a pacemaker

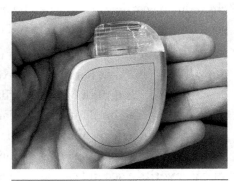

an implantable cardiac defibrillator

recover as much as possible. If, after that time, there remains a significant amount of unviable heart muscle and there is an ejection fraction around 30 percent or less, compelling data suggest that an implantable cardiac defibrillator could be inserted into these patients as a **primary** preventative measure. Research shows that these patients are at very high risk of having a life-threatening rhythm ('cardiac arrest') and it is better to put in a defibrillator **before** they have a problem rather than wait until after as they may not have another chance.

Although the data supporting primary prevention is compelling for patients who have had a large amount of heart muscle killed from lack of blood supply, the case doesn't seem to be as clear in terms of benefit for patients with non-ischemic cardiomyopathy.

This primary prevention strategy is highly specialized, and any decision often requires the input of a team of specialists.

Very important. In primary prevention, the worse the ejection fraction, the greater the benefit is likely to be to the patient. As the ejection fraction improves, the benefit of one of these devices becomes less.

resynchronization

Symptoms, heart function and mortality can also be improved in certain patients who have an abnormality in the way electrical impulses pass through the heart. A particular type of pacemaker, **a bi-ventricular pacemaker**, can improve the outcome for patients who have

- a significant reduction in their ejection fraction, less than about 35 percent, and

- an electrical abnormality of the heart, so that there is a discordant contraction of the heart.

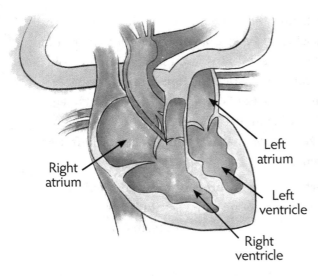

Right
atrium

Left
atrium

Left
ventricle

Right
ventricle

chambers of the heart

As we know, the heart has four chambers: the right atrium, left atrium, right ventricle, and left ventricle. Here, however, our focus is on the main pumping chamber of the heart, the left ventricle (LV). In a normal heart, the LV is electrically activated through the Purkinje fibers – special cells acting like wires within the heart – so that the compression is synchronous and coordinated. If there is a delay in the even distribution of the de-polarization signal – that is, a delay in the electrical impulse arriving in the left side of the LV so that the right side of the LV contracts and the left side contracts **after** the right – there is a problem.

To help understand this, visualize that you are holding a piano accordion or a squeezebox. It works as it was designed if the left hand and the right hand are coming together and pulling apart at the same time. If, however, the hands are not synchronous, and one hand works and then is followed by the other, the squeezebox is pushed rather than squeezed. An unexpected and unpleasant noise results because the instrument is not working as it should.

In the heart, if the timing in contraction is disrupted, such that one side of the heart activates followed by the other, then the contraction force, or efficiency, is diminished, just like the accordion. So, by putting small wires into the heart to deliver electrical impulses, both sides of the left ventricle can be activated at the same time, and the beautiful synchronicity of nature is re-established. Our 'accordion' is back 'in accord'.

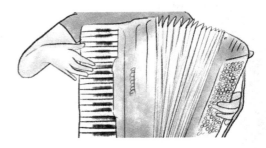

The use of these special pacemakers is called **resynchronization therapy**. These pacemakers work best in patients in whom

- maximum oral drug therapy has been used

- the ejection fraction is reduced to around 35 percent or less and

- there is a clear delay between electrical activation through the ventricle. That is measured from the ECG and is called the QRS width. If that QRS width is 150 milliseconds or greater, then there is very good data that cardiac resynchronization therapy is likely to be beneficial. This broadening of the QRS is called a bundle branch block. (Remember Martin?)

Resynchronization therapy not only improves symptoms, function and quality of life, it also improves outcome. As with the implantable cardiac defibrillator, this is a highly specialized area and requires specialist decision-making.

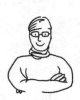

These specialized pacemakers can also be incorporated with an implantable cardiac defibrillator. The patient can have resynchronization to re-establish coordination of the heart contractions and also have a backup if a life-saving electrical shock is required. What amazing technology!

CASE STUDY – BARRY

shortness of breath, damaged lungs, enlarged heart, left bundle branch block, HFrEF, implantation of biventricular pacemaker

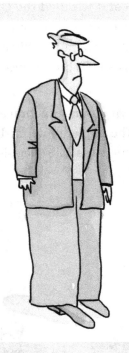

Barry was about 70 years old when we met in 2009. He was a natural joker who always had something funny to say. Unfortunately, at that time, life was not very funny for Bazza.

He had endured about 12 months of worsening shortness of breath, particularly on exertion, although he had not experienced any chest pain. (Chest pain could point to angina or narrowed or blocked arteries.) He had been a prolific smoker, and so his lungs were not healthy. Although he had given up smoking, the damage had been done. At the time, because of his smoking history, a respiratory (or lung) doctor was looking after him.

An x-ray showed that Barry had an enlarged heart. An electrocardiogram (ECG) showed an abnormally broad pattern in the QRS complex, which indicated a left bundle branch block (the left branch of the heart's electrical system was partially or wholly blocked causing the left ventricle to contract a little later than it should). A subsequent echocardiogram showed an ejection fraction of 28 percent, which was not good. (Remember, normal should be around 60 percent, so this was about half of normal.)

I became involved at that stage to help with heart failure with reduced ejection fraction (HFrEF).

An ACE inhibitor administered immediately helped. We also performed an invasive angiogram to check for any blockages or narrowing of the

heart's arteries. While we didn't find any blockages, there were some irregularities. So, I started Barry on a low dose of aspirin and some cholesterol-lowering medication to off-set any future risk of blocked arteries. He started intermittent diuretic therapy, which gave him some symptomatic improvement. He also began some beta-blocker, in his case, bisoprolol, starting at 1.25 milligrams for several weeks before increasing it to 2.5 mg and then, after some months, to 5 mg. Pleasingly, he started to feel better.

In 2013, with the use of up-titrated ACE inhibitor, up-titrated beta-blocker and the judicious use of diuretic therapy, Barry's ejection fraction had improved from 28 percent to between 30 and 35 percent. While this was a better reading, there was still room for improvement. There was space to increase the bisoprolol dose a little, so I did.

In 2015, having maximized his drug therapy, I wondered if, because of the bundle branch block, Barry could be a candidate for biventricular pacing (cardiac resynchronization). A promising and relatively new technology at that time, the procedure improves the left ventricle's ability to pump blood from the heart. Earlier that year, Barry had contracted influenza and had been hospitalized, very ill. While being monitored in a high-intensity unit, he recorded 16 beats of broad complex tachycardia, or ventricular tachycardia. Was it possible that Barry required a defibrillator? His ejection fraction had dropped to near 20 percent while he was in the hospital (pretty bad). When he was stable again, the possibility of biventricular pacing now included the addition of an implantable cardioverter-defibrillator. A colleague of mine in Melbourne undertook this procedure.

Six months later, an assessment of the implanted device showed that Barry was getting 97 percent of his beats coordinated through the biventricular pacemaker. This result ensured that both sides of the ventricle were receiving the electrical impulse simultaneously, coordinated contractions or 'an accordion in accord'. By March 2016, the ejection fraction had moved from about 20 percent to 25-30 percent. A year later, it had moved to 28-30 percent, and in January 2018, it was at 30-35 percent. And there it has remained.

Barry is now on maximum doses of ACE inhibitor and beta-blocker. The bi-ventricular pacemaker can de-fibrillate if it is required.

Barry has been through a lot during the past decade. He is as well as could be hoped for; he is functioning well and making the most of each day. He recently went on an overseas holiday and continues to have a new joke for me at each appointment.

Bazza was very ill with dys-synchrony from abnormal depolarization of the heart. He has benefited from bi-ventricular pacing and the implantation of a cardiac defibrillator that is capable of restoring rhythm to his heart should it be needed.

pulmonary artery blood pressure monitoring

Blood pressures in the pulmonary artery can be measured, although the technique is not commonly used. Tracking pressure within the pulmonary circulation gives a good indication of how pressures and blood flow could be loading the lungs and the heart. Adjustments to alter fluid balance can then be made to a patient's therapy. The aim is to keep the patient 'just right' in terms of

- not too much fluid, which could bring on shortness of breath, or a cough,

- nor too little fluid which could jeopardize the patient's kidney function, make the person lightheaded or lower the blood pressure.

While such monitoring is often used for critical and acute patients in intensive care units, the widespread use of the technology in outpatients has not been taken up yet as it requires that a small device be implanted into the pulmonary trunk, the short artery that transports carbon dioxide-rich blood from the right ventricle to the lungs.

cardiac contractility modulation

Cardiac contractility modulation is a relatively new implant technology that applies an electrical impulse to the heart at a particular stage within the cardiac cycle – during a particular stage of the ECG – that alters the way the calcium within the myocytes, the cells of the heart, is treated. This impulse increases the efficiency and the effectiveness of the contraction of the heart muscle. As well as altering calcium utilization, cardiac contractility modulation also alters phosphorylation, which is an energy-producing reaction within the cell, from beat to beat.

Cardiac contractility modulation can improve the way the heart beats with each pulse and, in the longer term, it can alter the way phosphorylation occurs within the cell, also improving outcomes. The therapy is particularly exciting for people who do not have the dissynchrony that responds well to resynchronization therapy. It is ideal for people with reduced ejection fraction (HFrEF) without delay in delivery of the electrical impulse into the left ventricle as shown by a narrow QRS complex.

The US Food and Drug Administration (FDA) has approved its use, and it is currently (2021) under review in other jurisdictions, including Australia. I don't have any patients using this technology. However, I look at it as an exciting opportunity. Time will tell where trial data go and where uptake and utilization lead us.

left atrium decompression

Another new intervention, **decompressing the left atrium**, is promising for patients who have heart failure with preserved ejection fraction (HFpEF). This type of cardiac failure is challenging to manage. Research on HFpEF cardiac failure shows that the pressure in the left atrium generally increases, and that pressure is then transmitted backwards into the lungs and forward into the left ventricle. So, researchers have been asking:

- can we decompress the left atrium?
- can we take pressure out of the system?
- can we reduce the pressure on the lungs and the left ventricle?

In trying to answer these questions, interesting research suggests that a hole could be made between the left atrium and the right atrium so that the blood drains from the left side to the right side, thus decompressing the left atrium. While it looks as if this may be a promising intervention, there is not much data yet, and so it is currently not standard practice.

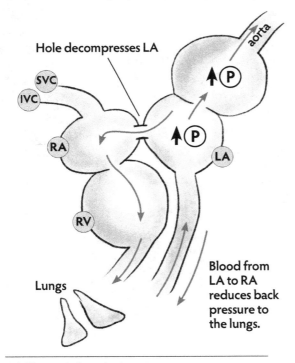

There is no question. Left atrium decompression is a really interesting space. Fancy making a hole in the heart to fix it!?!?

a deliberate hole in the heart?

restoring blood flow to viable tissue

For those patients who have developed cardiac failure because of coronary artery disease, or lack of blood flow to the heart, then **restoring blood flow** to viable tissue, that is, the tissue that is still alive, is a necessary therapy that produces good results.

Blood flow can be improved by

- inserting stents to open narrowings or blockages where appropriate, or

- undertaking bypass grafting.

The latter is where a piece of 'tube', from an artery or vein, takes blood around the blockage/s to a healthier artery so that good blood flow reaches the heart muscle. The catch here is that if inadequate blood supply damages the muscle, that part of the heart may have died, and the result is scar tissue.

No matter how much blood gets to dead tissue, it cannot be anything more than a scar because the tissue is no longer viable. There is no point in getting extra blood flow to an area of dead scar tissue as it simply won't help the patient.

Assessment of patients who have cardiac failure from coronary artery disease needs time. An evaluation of the area that needs blood, either via stent or via bypass, has to be made to determine if the muscle is still alive so that, if it again can receive good blood flow, it will recover and help the patient in the longer term. If good blood flow can be returned to viable tissue, it improves symptoms, as well as morbidity and mortality prospects for the patient.

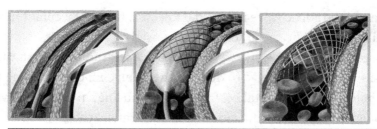

inserting a stent

valves

Failing heart valves give rise to failing hearts.

On the left side of the heart are the **mitral** valve and the **aortic** valve. When either valve becomes too tight, this is called **stenosis**. When either valve is leaking, it is called **regurgitation** (or incompetence). Either way and with either valve, the heart can end up in failure.

mitral valve

Most commonly, a severe problem with the mitral valve, either not opening or leaking, results in surgery where the valve can be either repaired or replaced. Ideally, if the patient's valve is suitable, the repair is the best outcome. If a replacement valve is to be used, then a discussion among the patient, the cardiologist and the surgeon is generally undertaken. Whether the replacement valve is made of metallic or biological tissue depends on the specific needs of the patient. The correct valve selection assures the best solution.

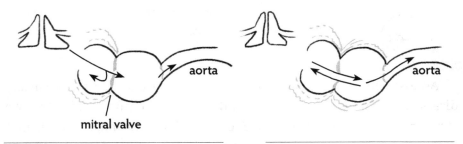

mitral stenosis: all of the blood does not pass through the valve, and the atrium dilates

mitral incompetence: blood leaks back through the valve, and the atrium and ventricle dilate

aortic valve

Rarely is the aortic valve repaired. However, two replacement methods are available. Open heart surgery has been used for many years. Now, there is also a relatively new technology that passes a wire and a balloon catheter to the site of the aortic valve to deploy a new valve made of natural tissue that is held open by a metal scaffold. This amazing, minimally invasive, technology is called a **t**ranscutaneous (or **t**ranscatheter) **a**ortic **v**alve implantation or **TAVI**.

The TAVI procedure is generally **not** used for:

- people who need surgery for their arteries at the same time, as there is no point in performing a minimally invasive valve procedure when the chest is being opened to deal with the arteries, or

- patients who have a leaky valve, as it just does not seem to work as well.

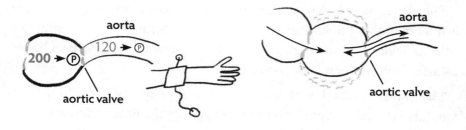

aortic stenosis: blood is forced through a narrowed valve, and the ventricle thickens in response

aortic incompetence: blood leaks back into the ventricle

Choice of the valve is a complex, changing and patient-specific consideration.

In general terms, metallic valves last longer. While there is no surprise there, they come at a cost. The patient needs to take a blood thinner (such as warfarin, an anticoagulant that requires regular blood test monitoring) for life. The blood thinner will lower the risk of a clot forming on the valve. Such a clot could stop the valve from working or the clot could break off and go to the brain, causing a stroke.

In comparison, tissue valves generally do not require blood thinners (anticoagulation) and so are 'easier to live with' for the patient. They tend to have a lower risk of becoming infected but can wear out, particularly in younger patients, and so may mean a second procedure.

heart transplant

For some patients, a heart transplant, where the patient is given a new heart from a donor, is a final option. Specialists in dedicated units perform heart transplants. As part of the process, very specific, detailed attention is given to patient selection and donor management by a team of experts who work extensively in this arena.

The sickest people who are not responding to other therapies are the recipients of this life-changing technology. Generally, they are younger patients who tend not to have other medical issues and whose life is sustainable until a new heart is available.

The main drawback is that the number of people who could benefit from this medical miracle far outnumbers the availability of donor hearts. Although it is a tremendous procedure for an excellent therapeutic opportunity and an amazing way to turn someone's life around, it is also a situation where you don't wish for donors because of the sadness on that side of the story.

Another exciting and extensive area of work is trying to raise pigs with tissue markers that would allow transplant into a human without rejection. This procedure is called a **xenograft**, and, if achievable, would address the supply issue.

A heart transplant is an incredible intervention which is supported with particular medications and by particular specialist units of medical caregivers who have a high degree of specialty in this space. After two to three decades of using this procedure, people now survive for many, many years and lead near-normal lives. It is incredible to think that someone else's beating heart could save another life.

left ventricular assist device

Patients who are suitable for transplant and are in the end stages of heart failure can be kept alive with a **left ventricular assist device** (LVAD).

Such a device is a pump piggybacked on to the heart using surgical techniques.

The LVAD usually has an external component that holds the battery and provides the power for the unit. The pump works in conjunction with the patient's own heart to keep blood pressure stabilized and blood flowing. This keeps the patient alive for weeks to months, hopefully until an appropriate donor becomes available.

Incredible, fantastic technology! Incredible in the way it can save lives and fantastic for the difference it can make to a person's life.

GORDON'S JOURNEY

the gift of life

I had my heart attack in 1992. I was aged 37. After time in an intensive care unit (ICU) in Hobart, I had two balloons inserted into clogged arteries to try to unblock them (a procedure called angioplasty[9]).

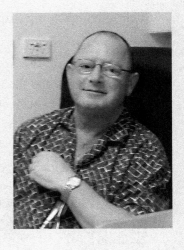

In 1995, I underwent a bypass. After the operation, the surgeon said if he had known how badly my heart was damaged, he possibly wouldn't have attempted the bypass. For the next 10 years, I worked, and my heart worked, and I had no real problems.

Then, in 2005, a carotid artery almost completely blocked. That's the artery taking blood to the brain, so I was lucky. I didn't have any side-effects from the surgery. My heart wasn't right, though, so I needed to have a pacemaker and defibrillator installed. The pacemaker resynchronized the coordination of the electrical impulse in the heart and if my heart really 'played up' and stopped, the defibrillator would shock it back into rhythm. This time my luck didn't hold, and there were complications. I underwent an operation where the surgeon used a da Vinci robot – I'm not sure why he used this minimally-invasive surgical method, but I think it was to be more precise with finer movements – and, again, I ended up in ICU.

On recovery, my cardiologist continued to monitor my health regularly. Over several years, several stents were inserted into my arteries. This was on top of the initial balloons and subsequent to the bypass. Then, in 2011, he said, "It's time for a new heart", and referred me to the heart transplant clinic at a major hospital in Melbourne, the Alfred Hospital[10].

I attended a five-day assessment where the doctors checked me for everything. It was interesting in that I needed to be sick enough to require a new heart but healthy enough to receive one. A challenging balance.

Following the assessment, I was told that I wouldn't benefit from a heart transplant at that time; however, they would retain me on their books. I was delighted. I thought, "Right, I'm going to be alright!" but it was short-lived.

Fortunately for me, I had my implanted defibrillator. It activated on two occasions. The second time, it needed three 'goes' to 'get me right' — and it saved my life. It was mid-2012 by now, and the heart transplant team decided to put me on the waiting list for a new heart. The phone call came in July 2013. Well, what an experience! I received a phone call from the Heart Transplant Coordinator on a Saturday. Some conversations you just don't forget.

He said, "Great news, Gordon, we have a heart for you. Can you be here by 12 o'clock?"

I said, "Yes. I'll ring the airlines", and I hung up.

After several calls, it was impossible to get a flight out of Hobart, so I called him back.

"No problems. I will send the Air Ambulance."

At the airport, the paramedic explained that the weather in Melbourne was bad and he might not be able to land the aircraft. There was another option. A Qantas jet was being held on the tarmac, and it had two first-class seats available. Finally, a Qantas medical doctor in Sydney gave permission for me to be transported. On boarding the aircraft, the passengers all cheered! Then, when I got off, they all sang out, "Good luck!" It was 11:20 am.

It was raining very heavily, and the ambulance driver sat me up straight as we 'flew' down Tullamarine Freeway on our way to the hospital. It was a scary ride.

When we arrived at The Alfred, I was rushed to the operating area. 11:45 am. Everything happened so quickly. Now, it's about seven minutes to midday. Usually, it can take up to two hours to check compatibility. I was there only minutes before they announced it matched and the anesthetist said, "See you soon".

I woke with a tube down my throat and a nurse by my side. I felt as if I'd just been through hell. After three days, I was sitting up in bed feeling a million bucks, thinking, "This is a breeze. I'm going to live forever!" Then, a couple of days later while still in ICU, I had a bad turn. Luckily for me, the nurse was there. The team rushed in and gave me medication. I came good, eventually.

After being moved from the ICU but still on the cardiovascular ward, I awoke suddenly one night to find several people around me saying, "Stay with me, mate! Stay with me, mate! You'll be right. Stay with me, mate!" Little did I know that I was on death's door again. With their professionalism and skill, they saved me.

After about 12 days, I was discharged to a unit in Melbourne. I was to call it 'home' for the next six months.

However, that first night, suddenly, fluid started leaking from where they had taken out the drains. I was rushed back to the hospital. I had an infection which took weeks to clear. Eventually, I returned to the unit to recuperate, going daily to the hospital for rehabilitation and exercise. By November-early December I was able to travel back to Hobart.

While recovering and although still on some medication, my breastbone was not healing. It was always moving, and I was not feeling very well.

I went back to The Alfred, and they decided to operate. They found poison, an infection, in the chest, and this was not allowing the bone to heal. I spent another month in the hospital and underwent several operations in which they tried to clean the bone and fight the infection. Eventually, a flap operation[11] was performed on my chest, and, finally, I went home to Hobart.

After two months of having an antibiotic drip in my arm full-time, and numerous trips to the Royal Hobart Hospital (RHH), my chest was

This is a painful situation. The rib cage needs to be stable so that when the diaphragm moves up and down the chest does not collapse in on itself. Gordon's situation was made worse as lack of healing was caused by an infection. Remember, the immune-suppressive agents used to prevent rejection can increase the chance of infection.

186

still moving, and I was in agony. So, back again to The Alfred; this time to try to rewire me back up and to ensure the infection was coming under control. Another three weeks in the hospital, and again more infection. Eventually, I was transferred to the RHH where I stayed in the infectious disease ward for some time. Then, another six months of antibiotics being constantly dripped into me.

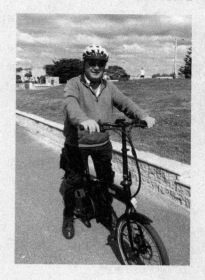

I came good.   It had taken about 18 months.

Apart from the physical journey that I have described, the mental trauma was significant. As part of the preparation for my heart transplant, I saw a psychiatrist, needing an assessment to confirm that I could mentally handle such an operation.

There are so many thoughts going through your mind before and after; things like,

- *will I survive,*
- *will I be better,*
- *will it be painful*

and after

- *how lucky was I,*
- *did I deserve it,*
- *what about the donor and that person's family?*

How can I ever thank the donor and the family for the gift of life?

People often ask me if I feel any different.

Yes, I do. I have somebody else's heart. That person, in life, had a family, went to school, had a career and things to look forward to. I often think about such things.

People ask me if I have changed, as, physically, I look the same.

Yeah, I do look the same, but inside I'm different. My values, my thoughts, my ambitions have all changed. Material things mean little to me, now. I am more emotional, and I feel quite different. It's hard to explain.

One thing that I do know, though, is someone gave me the gift life. And to that person, I say, "Thank you". ♥

The world's first human heart transplant was performed at Groote Schuur Hospital, Cape Town, South Africa, by surgeon Christiaan Barnard, on 3 December 1967. The 'new' heart functioned normally until the recipient's death from double pneumonia 18 days after the historic operation.

The first Australian heart transplant was performed in 1968 at St Vincent's Hospital, Sydney. Heart transplants have been performed regularly in Australia since 1984. Heart transplant centers are in Sydney, Melbourne, Brisbane and Perth.

At the end of 2006, more than 74,000 heart, 2800 heart-lung, 7300 single lung and 6000 bilateral lung transplants had been performed worldwide.[12] Worldwide, the overall survival rate is more than 85 percent after one year and about 69 percent after five years for adults, despite an increase in older and higher risk transplant recipients.[13]

---

[9] In the early days of angioplasty, balloons only were used to open the clogged artery. Today, when angioplasty is employed, it can be with or without the addition of a stent, a wire mesh scaffold which decreases the chance of the artery narrowing again.

[10] "The Alfred", the Alfred Hospital, in Melbourne, Australia, provides specialty services in a number of treatments, including cardiology. It is a leading tertiary hospital (associated with Monash University) and houses the largest intensive care unit in Australia. In 1957, The Alfred was the first hospital in Australia to place a patient on a cardiopulmonary bypass to treat complex cardiac lesions.

[11] Flap surgery involves transporting healthy, live tissue (with an intact blood supply) from one location of the body to another. This is not a graft, which does not have a blood supply.

[12] https://www.heartfoundation.org.au/images/uploads/publications/Heart-Transplants-Donations.pdf

[13] https://www.mayoclinic.org/tests-procedures/heart-transplant/about/pac-20384750

CF patients can be helped beyond medications through a variety of implantable devices and/or surgical procedures:

- **implantable cardiac defibrillator**
  - provides constant monitoring for several years
  - 'shocks' the patient back into life should the patient 'die'

- **resynchronization therapy**
  - uses a bi-ventricular pacemaker to synchronize the heart's electrical impulses

- **pulmonary artery BP monitoring**
  - tracks pressure within the pulmonary circulation to indicate pressures and flow in the heart and lungs

- **cardiac contractility modulation**
  - increases the efficiency and effectiveness of the contraction of the muscle of the heart

- **left atrium decompression**
  - new research suggests that a hole could be made between the left and right atria so that blood flows from the left side to the right side (not current practice)

- **restoring blood flow to viable tissue**
  - inserting stents or bypass grafts for patients with coronary artery disease achieve good results

(continued next page)

- **valves**
  - mitral, tight or leaking, needs surgery
    - replaced (with biological or metallic tissue) or
    - repaired
  - aortic, two methods of replacement
    - open heart surgery
    - TAVI, transcutaneous aortic valve implantation
- **heart transplant**
  - a heart from a donor
  - for the sickest patients
    - often young without other health issues
    - whose life can be sustained until a new heart is available
  - number of potential recipients far outweighs number of donors
    - xenograft, using pig tissue, is being studied as a potential source
- **ventricular assist device**
  - external pump that works in conjunction with the patient's own heart until a heart from a donor is available

Treatment of cardiac failure goes hand-in-glove with the treatment of its common partners.

chapter 16
COMMON PARTNERS

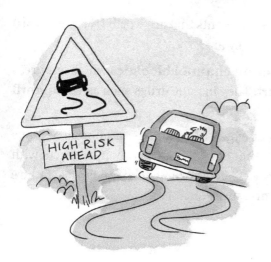

Cardiac failure has common partners in several other medical disorders. High blood pressure, atrial fibrillation, coronary heart disease, diabetes, obesity, sleep apnea, aging, anemia, and cancer can link to cardiac failure. In most cases, these conditions are **associations** rather than causations of the problem; they **contribute to**, rather than initiate, cardiac failure.

An easy way to understand these concepts of association and causation is to think of a traffic accident. Speeding and alcohol consumption are significant associations of car accidents. However, people drive over the speed limit with a high alcohol level and do not have accidents. People who have not been drinking can drive within the speed limit and still have an accident. Neither the speeding nor alcohol **causes** the car accident; speeding and alcohol do not drive the car. Yet, they **contribute** to the accident. They are **associations**. Multiple associations such as alcohol, speeding, driving experience, and weather can be factors in one accident. The actual cause of the accident might be a dog running out onto the street, the driver losing concentration, a car in front stops suddenly.

CF associations add to the 'wear and tear' on the heart, are often **precursors** to the failure and must be treated in connection with the cardiac failure.

blood pressure

Blood pressure is linked to the development of cardiac failure. Agents such as the ACE inhibitors, angiotensin receptor blockers, beta-blockers, aldosterone blockers, and the neprilysin blockers **work very well** for heart failure. They also all regulate blood pressure.

However, there are blood pressure agents that are worth trying to **avoid** in the presence of cardiac failure. They are:

- the **centrally-acting calcium channel blockers** which suppress the contractility of the heart. They include drugs such as **verapamil** and **diltiazem**,

- the drug, **moxonidine** that works through the autonomic nervous system. Research suggests that because of the way it interacts with the autonomic nervous system, it is not beneficial for cardiac failure although useful for blood pressure control.

atrial fibrillation

Another common companion is atrial fibrillation (AF). When the heart's top chambers, the atria, are not pumping correctly, the pump loses its efficiency. The situation compounds if someone who already has cardiac failure goes into atrial fibrillation.

The recent CASTLE AF trial[14] looked at patients with poor heart function with ejection fractions of about 35 percent or less who had intermittent runs of AF. Patients were randomized into a group who had undergone electrophysiological (EP) ablation[15] of their AF and another group who were on standard care. The trial showed that the EP ablation group had better outcomes in terms of mortality, morbidity, and hospitalization.

An improved pump should result in a better outcome for the patient. If, however, the patient cannot be brought out of AF and has cardiac failure, then the risk of stroke is very, very high. There is no question that these patients will benefit from anticoagulation to reduce the risk of clot formation and potential stroke. [16]

CASE STUDY – CHARLIE

atrial flutter, severe LV dysfunction, HFrEF, tachycardia-induced cardiomyopathy

Charlie didn't think he had cardiac failure. He was an active and fit 84-year-old man when I was asked to see him. He had been prepped and was ready for orthopedic surgery to replace his hip when a very rapid heartbeat was detected. His heart rate was well over 100 beats a minute. I was called by the anesthetist to see if the surgery should go ahead.

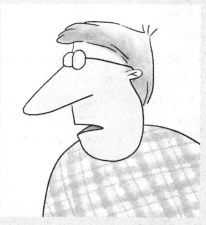

Charlie had atrial flutter, a rapid and regular rhythm arising from the right side of the heart. As Charlie's surgery was elective, we decided to delay the operation so I could explore further what was happening with his heart to stabilize the situation.

Amazingly, Charlie had very little in the way of symptoms. He was a bit grumpy with me that I had canceled the surgery that, quite reasonably, he wanted to have behind him. He was hemodynamically (hemodynamic, the dynamics of blood flow) stable. Although his heart rate was up, his blood pressure was not too bad and he was able to stand and walk around. He didn't have a significant postural drop and he was relatively functional. So, apart from his heart racing, he seemed in pretty good shape.

Because of his atrial flutter, we did an echocardiogram to see how the left ventricle was pumping and how the chamber looked. Surprisingly, he had severe left ventricular

Atrial flutter is similar to the 'irregularly irregular' AF but is a more 'organized' rhythm.

dysfunction. His ejection fraction was 25 percent (remember, normal ejection fraction is about 60 percent).

...
Good thing we canceled the surgery!
...

Immediately, I put a therapy regime in place to help a heart that was not working properly. I commenced Charlie on an ACE inhibitor (and watched his blood pressure), a beta-blocker (and watched his blood pressure), and some digoxin to help slow down his heart and control the atrial flutter. We increased the beta-blocker slowly because it is known to slow the rate of atrial flutter as well. I also started Charlie on a blood-thinning medication to reduce the risk of a clot forming in the atrium.

The seriousness of atrial flutter is that it carries the risk of a clot forming in the person's heart. That clot can break away and make its way to the brain, causing a stroke. BAD. We want to mitigate that risk as best as possible.

Some weeks later, I saw Charlie again.

His heart rate was down to 50+ beats a minute. The digoxin, which was helping with rate control, was in the therapeutic range. The beta-blocker, which was dampening the sympathetic nervous system and helping to control the rate and protect his heart, was being well-tolerated, and the ACE inhibitor was being up-titrated. We repeated the echocardiogram, and his ejection fraction had gone from 25 to 50 percent. And so, I sent him off for his surgery.

The good thing about the change in Charlie's ejection fraction was that it showed that his heart failure was reversible. His repeat echocardiogram pointed to the most likely cause of the problem being that his heart had been beating too fast for too long. This is called tachycardia (fast heart rate) induced (causing) cardiomyopathy (cardio – heart; myo – muscle; opathy

– problem). As seen in Charlie's case, correcting tachycardia can reverse tachycardia-induced cardiomyopathy and so restore heart function.

When I saw Charlie over those months before his surgery, he was fairly adamant that he had little in the way of symptoms and was still upset that I had postponed the surgery. Somewhat begrudgingly, he was taking his medications.

I saw Charlie late in 2019 for a two-year follow-up. Pleasingly, his ejection fraction was at 55 percent, which is within the normal range. He was still denying problems. This time, however, it is fair to say that he probably didn't have any problems!

I'm pleased to say, also, he was still taking his medications. Good news. We know that if we lose control of his heart rate, the tachycardia-induced cardiomyopathy could come back and we also know that maintaining those medications, in the longer term, is a sensible idea.

Charlie has done well, albeit with some delay to his orthopedic surgery, and, interestingly, for someone who, from the beginning, really didn't describe much in the way of symptoms. A great outcome for a very interesting case.

Too many patients stop taking their medications because, down the track, they 'feel better'. They think they don't need them anymore — until they end up back in the hospital or worse. Most heart medications do not have an end-point where the condition has been cured. For CF patients, consistently taking the medication is a life-improving, long-term commitment.

coronary artery disease

Nearly 50 percent of all patients with CF have some coronary artery disease (CAD), a build-up of plaque in the artery that leads to a narrowing of the artery and reduced blood flow. A complication is that a CAD symptom can be shortness of breath as an angina variant.

Although 'angina' describes the pain associated with lack of blood to the heart muscle, it also can present as shortness of breath.

If the heart receives inadequate blood, say, during exercise, the heart muscle cramps. The pain of 'angina' is really the pain of the heart muscle cramping. Sometimes, the cramp does not give rise to pain and, instead, the individual suffers the consequence of the heart not working properly. The cramped muscle is stiff and does not relax as blood flows into it. This increases pressures within the heart which are transmitted to the lungs, leading to congestion and difficulty in breathing. So, shortness of breath becomes an 'angina' equivalent or variant.

The doctor must determine if the person has shortness of breath because of poor arteries or if inadequate management of cardiac failure is the driver. Sometimes, a functional test, such as a treadmill test (stress test), can be a useful start to the investigation as it shows clear evidence that the heart is not receiving enough blood. In this case, the shortness of breath indicates problems in the arteries.

Remember, it could be both.

A blood test to check brain natriuretic peptide levels is another way to determine the cause. Extremely high levels of this peptide indicate that the heart is under strain and probably failing, and so the shortness of breath can be attributed to cardiac failure.

diabetes

One group of diabetes agents, **glitazones**, has been shown to increase the likelihood of CF. These tablets cause the body to hold fluid, thus throwing out the individual's fluid balance. However, as we have already learnt, it is not all bad news for people with diabetes who need to manage their sugar and CF. The sodium-glucose transport inhibitors, SGLT2 blockers, help to control sugar levels by allowing sugar to pass out through the urine. As mentioned earlier, a relatively recent trial[17] (2016), the EMPA-REG OUTCOME trial, which looked at the medication empagliflozin and was designed principally for diabetes management, showed an impressive reduction in cardiac failure complications in the treatment group.

The 2016 EMPA-REG OUTCOME trial result[17] really raised eyebrows and has brought an incredible focus to this group of drugs. Numerous studies are currently underway, trying to understand better how these agents may work in cardiac failure more broadly.

SGLT2 inhibitors block the exchange of sodium and glucose within the kidney, making the patient pass a little bit more urine containing sodium and glucose. Remember, renal disease can be a common association of CF as well. This is partly because the diuretics used can shut down renal function, either accidentally or if patients need to be 'dried out' for their heart failure. The autonomic drive is also trying to constrict blood vessels while maintaining kidney function.

Have you ever noticed that if you are stressed – perhaps before a job interview, exam or public speaking – you often feel a nature call to empty your bladder?

obesity

The heart of an overweight person with CF is going to do more work than is needed. Obesity, which is certainly linked to cardiac failure, needs addressing, and as early as possible.

asthma

Asthma is a common condition and can be a companion to cardiac failure. Because both CF and asthma give rise to shortness of breath, it is important to determine which is the dominant problem for the patient at any given time.

sleep apnea

Patients with CF have altered central breathing. As well as the other problems cardiac failure patients have, their respiratory center, the area in the brain that sets the rate and depth of breathing, is affected, and becomes less effective. This means CF patients may breathe at a variant rate, particularly while they are asleep. The breathing can be shallow and then deep, while the rate speeds up or slows down. That variant rate breathing does not respond well to the positive pressure ventilation used by a person who has obstructive sleep apnea.

Patients who have obstructive sleep apnea as well as CF, however, need to be assessed appropriately as their daily sense of wellbeing and, of course, their energy levels benefit from obstructive sleep apnea treatment. The caution here is that the ventilator devices can cause more harm than good if used in the wrong situations.

ageing

As CF is more common in the older population, many patients also suffer from gout and arthritis. Nonsteroidal anti-inflammatory drugs (NSAIDs) and COX-2 inhibitor drugs, used for pain relief in the treatment of arthritis, can shut down the kidney and are linked to fluid retention. Their use needs to be sparing and careful. *(refer back to our earlier discussion on NSAIDs, pages 151-153)*

the psychological aspects associated with cardiac failure

The other illnesses that we talk about in this chapter can **contribute to** cardiac failure. Depression is a common partner in that it **results from** cardiac failure. Twenty percent of patients with cardiac failure suffer from depression. Recognizing depression is fundamental for a person's quality of life. It is crucial also to cardiac failure outcome, mortality and mobility since depression has recognized cardiovascular risk implications. Medical practitioners need to be aware that **depression is an association of cardiac failure**, and they need to be ready to treat it, if necessary.

CF is a serious and long-term condition. So, it is not hard to imagine that people dealing with either acute or chronic CF are also dealing with a significant impact on their daily lives. CF symptoms bring on feelings of uncertainty, and, potentially, fear and anxiety, followed by investigations by doctors whom the patients are not used to seeing. This experience culminates in being given a diagnosis of CF – a confronting and scary situation that calls for empathy.

As well as dealing with their CF symptoms that affect them daily, one in five CF patients needs to deal with **mood alteration**, which adds another, significant impact to each day. Studies show that the patients who have been hospitalized due to their CF have a higher rate of depression compared with out-patients. This finding makes sense. The more ill people are, the more likely they are to find themselves in hospital, and the more likely they are to be afraid, aware of the potential impact on their life and well-being, and ultimately on their mortality. Importantly, however, depression for individuals with cardiac failure is associated with a worse prognosis, which is reduced life expectancy or admissions to hospital.

Doctors, patients and carers need to be aware of the possibility of depression with CF. Doctors need to tune in to a patient's needs. Patients should be told that they are allowed to feel 'down' about what is going on. However, they also need to be able to recognize if they are 'down' more than they should be for what appears to be happening in their lives. This is an important flag, too, of which carers and others close to the patient should be aware.

Screening tools are available, such as the Patient Health Questionnaire (PHQ). If there is any uncertainly about the presence of depression in the setting of cardiac failure, CF patients should ask their GP to take them through it. Often, it can be the patient's partner who raises it with the doctor, a very good reason for patients to attend appointments with their 'important other'.

Research data show that:

- **cognitive behavioral therapy** – how our thinking drives our behavior and how changed thinking can change behavior – can be beneficial for treating depression associated with CF;

- meta-analysis based on studies involving **exercise** for CF sufferers has shown it to be beneficial for mood;

- joining groups of people with similar problems, enjoying nature, taking up a hobby, socializing, are further **life-style changes** that can help combat depression, and

- in comparison to the above beneficial therapies to combat depression in the setting of CF, work has shown that **anti-depressant drugs** – the selective serotonin-reuptake inhibitors (SSRIs) and, in particular, escitalopram and sertraline – were as equally effective as a placebo, meaning, they had **no effect**.

Please exercise and undertake more activities to keep your happy hormones high!

- CF is very common in today's society
- depression in CF sufferers is common – about 20 percent
  - worsening CF prognosis, and
  - worsening quality of life
- research shows that for depression in the setting of CF
  - cognitive behavioral therapy is helpful
  - anti-depressant drugs are **not** helpful
  - exercise is fantastic
- if you are
  - **suffering CF**, talk with your GP and have a self-audit (PHQ)
  - **caring for someone** with CF, ensure the person is traveling as well as he or she can be, and
  - **a doctor caring for CF patients**, keep depression front-of-mind

anemia

If anemia is discovered with CF, reversible causes such as loss of blood from the gut are sought.

A hormone produced by the kidneys to stimulate the production of red blood cells, **erythropoietin**, commonly known as EPO, should **not** be used as a treatment. While its use as a performance enhancer can bring about the disqualification of a Tour de France cyclist, in a CF patient, stimulating red blood cell growth can lead to increased clotting – a **problem**.

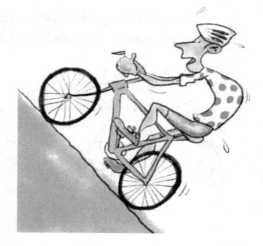

iron

The body's metabolism changes with CF and this can affect the way iron is stored. Up to 50 percent of patients have depleted iron reserves. These levels need to be tracked using a blood test that measures ferritin, a blood protein that contains iron, and, if low, the iron needs to be replenished. Having a decent steak will not do it, however. CF patients with low iron levels need to receive the iron through the vein. This markedly improves the way the patient feels and also improves the functional capacity of the heart.

cancer

A number of chemotherapeutic medications can harm the heart and can lead to CF, either acutely or delayed. The concern here is for patients who may currently be going through chemotherapy or who have already received treatment for cancer. Factors include the type of cancer and, therefore, the agents used, the set of treatment cycles, and the age of the patient.

Before chemotherapy, depending on the agent(s) being used, cancer patients will have their hearts checked using ultrasound and the results will be recorded in order to document a baseline for their heart health. Then, during chemotherapy, the oncologist who is administering the therapy should monitor, as appropriate, for any significant changes in heart function.

Should a patient present later with an abnormality of heart function, the baseline measurement and the chemotherapy history are imperative.

While breast cancer treatment is particularly significant, CF concern applies to all cancer treatments.

Several common partners contribute to, rather than cause, CF. They are:

blood pressure

- needs control;
- some BP medications work well in a CF setting, others should be avoided

atrial fibrillation

- needs control;
- otherwise, the risk of stroke is very high;

ageing

- pain relief drugs should be used sparingly and with caution

depression

- has cardio risk implications

anemia

- reversible causes are sought,
- do not treat with EPO

iron

- 50 percent of CF patients have depleted reserves;
- treatment is through the vein, not orally, with marked improvement to heart and wellbeing

cancer

- chemotherapeutic medications can lead to CF, either soon after treatment, or delayed
- chemotherapy history is important.

[14]   CASTLE-AF trial (Catheter Ablation for Atrial Fibrillation with Heart Failure) New
        England Journal of Medicine 2018; 378:417-427
        https://www.nejm.org/doi/full/10.1056/NEJMoa1707855

[15]   electrophysiological ablation is a method used to restore and maintain sinus rhythm
        within the heart. Is a highly specialized technique performed in only some cardiac units,
        when lifestyle modifications and drug therapies do not effectively control symptomatic
        atrial fibrillation

[16]   for a detailed discussion of AF, see my previous book, Atrial Fibrillation Explained (2019)

[17]   op. cit. Empagliflozin, Cardiovascular Outcomes

What happens when the heart fails suddenly?

chapter 17
ACUTE CARDIAC FAILURE

When a heart fails suddenly it is called acute cardiac failure. It is a medical emergency.

When a person presents with acute cardiac failure, the person has congestion. This build-up of fluid in the lungs gives rise to significant symptoms of **shortness of breath** and a **racing heart**. The body responds as if under stress, so

- the person sweats,

- the heart will be racing,

- the skin shuts down and it feels clammy,

This is cardiogenic shock, and it is life-threatening.

- blood pressure will have dropped, and often,

- the body won't be making much urine,

- the patient will be agitated and gasping for breath.

diagnosis

The diagnosis should be made as quickly as possible and often can be apparent from the clinical examination. The patient is unwell, clammy, short of breath with evidence of fluid loading and raised central pressure. The jugular venous pressure is visible in the neck and the patient is wheezing or making wet, rasping or crackling noises. Listening to the back of the lungs gives characteristic features of crackles. These crackles can be heard generally at the lower parts of the lungs although, sometimes, they can also be heard throughout the lungs. Swelling in the periphery, such as the legs, may also be evident, but necessarily in acute cardiac decompensation.

The presenting symptoms depend on the cause of the CF. Essentially, though, the doctor obtains history, examines the patient and organizes an

ECG. Almost invariably, a tachycardia (fast heart rhythm) or an abnormality of the heart muscle shows up and, so, points to the heart as the problem. As part of the work-up of shortness of breath, a chest x-ray could display fluid on the lungs but may also show an enlarged heart, again implicating the heart as the cause of this person's acute, serious presentation.

As a matter of urgency, the doctor organizes an ultrasound of the heart.

- How well is the heart muscle pumping?
- Is there a problem with the valves of the heart?

The ultrasound also measures pressures within the circulation, particularly within the lungs.

- Is there back pressure within the lungs due to poor function of the left ventricle?
- Have clots moved to the lungs and increased the resistance to blood passing through the lungs?

stabilization

Simultaneously with starting the diagnostic strategies, we aim to stabilize the patient as best as possible.

Lying the person down would distribute the congestion and decrease the efficiency of each breath.

Firstly, the patient **sits up** so that the congestion within the lungs drops to the bottom part of the lungs. This allows the top of the lungs to receive more oxygen, thus improving the efficiency of the lungs.

Next, **good intravenous access** is established so that bloods can be taken and drugs given. The blood work helps establish if there is anemia, an infection or electrolyte imbalance, and it can check for CF markers such as brain natriuretic peptides (BNP). High BNP supports the possibility that the person's heart is the problem. The troponin level can also be checked for stress on the heart. Troponin is a protein found in the heart that leaks into the bloodstream when the heart becomes stressed or damaged.

If the doctor believes it is CF, the patient often receives a small dose of the opiate, **morphine**, which helps lower anxiety. The morphine can also open up the blood vessels in a favorable way, particularly on the venous side of the circulation, reducing the amount of blood returning to the heart and lessening the heart's workload.

Your sympathetic drive is rarely your friend when your heart is playing up.

If the patient is low in oxygen, **supplementing oxygen** makes the person more comfortable; it also helps with oxygenating the tissues. Depending on how short of breath the person is, nasal specs or a mask deliver the extra oxygen. A ventilator with a mask that seals on to the face delivers more oxygen to the patient as the mask provides continuous positive airway pressure ventilation. This pushes air into the lungs at a higher pressure than the patient could achieve when breathing naturally. The extra air pushes fluid out of the lungs, which also changes the pressure within the chest cavity (thorax). A diminished gradient (difference) between the pressures inside and outside the thorax also decreases the heart's workload, and, as a consequence, the heart works better. Increased pressure in the thorax reduces the amount of venous return, also off-loading pressure on the heart.

The patient also receives **diuretics** through the vein as there may be reduced absorption through the gut during this time of sympathetic over-drive as blood diverts from the gut into other tissues. Typically, administering the loop-diuretic, furosemide, makes the patient pass urine to start off-loading the congestion.

Only if the person has **raised blood pressure** would blood pressure-lowering agents be administered. Vasodilators can take pressure off the heart if there is 'room to move' with the blood pressure.

If the blood pressure is too low, in very specific circumstances, the treating doctor may try to raise the blood pressure. Blood pressure that is too low is part of that cardiogenic shock symptom complex and could lead to not only renal failure but damage to other organs. The doctor might choose to trickle in a small quantity of drugs that mimic sympathetic drive to raise the blood pressure and make the heart pump more vigorously. These drugs are called **inotropes**. Essentially, they are adrenaline-type substances that may improve perfusion – the passage of fluid through the circulatory system to an organ or a tissue in the body. This is only an **acute strategy** and needs careful execution as, has been mentioned elsewhere, the sympathetic nervous system is not your friend if your heart is not working well.

highly specialized equipment

For people who are severely ill and who are in tertiary and quaternary referral centers – hospitals that have highly specialized equipment – there are several mechanical options available for treatment of CF.

One remarkable procedure, called **ultrafiltration**, sucks fluid out of the circulatory system using a process similar to dialysis. The patient's blood passes through a machine and less blood returns to the body. Ultrafiltration is an extraordinary way of taking fluid out of the body's circulation. It does not require drugs and does not need the kidneys to be functioning well. The difference between ultrafiltration and dialysis is that the latter also removes the body's waste products.

In an acute situation, specialist devices, which help the heart pump, can be implanted. A highly specific intervention is an **intra-aortic balloon pump** (IABP) for 'counter pulsation'. A balloon, placed in the aorta, expands and contracts, synchronized with the heartbeat. When the heart relaxes, the balloon expands to ensure the blood pressure is maintained, and when the heart is about to contract and release blood into the aorta, the balloon collapses, making it easier for the heart to pump. This fantastic piece of technology needs to be timed meticulously to that individual's heartbeat.

Another particular intervention for critically unwell patients whom specialists believe can be restored to a good quality of life, is **ECMO, e**xtra **c**orporeal **m**embrane **o**xygenation (*extra*, outside; *corporeal*, the body; *membrane*, the mechanism of exchange; *oxygen*, what is used). A machine, very similar to a by-pass machine (used in heart surgery to continue blood flow and perfusion to the body while the heart is immobilized as it is operated on), takes blood from the patient to enable a transfer of oxygen through a membrane outside the body to maintain oxygenation to the person.

As mentioned previously, there are also mechanical devices that 'piggyback' on to the heart and connect as support pumps. Left ventricular assist devices (LVAD) are implanted at a sub-acute stage to help support the circulation. These are generally used for patients whom it is believed will, in the future, undergo a heart transplant, or whose heart is likely to recover by itself.

causation

Stabilizing the patient is important when a person presents with acute CF. Another important aspect is ascertaining what caused the problem. If the problem is immediately reversible, an opportunity exists to make a big difference for the patient.

Most commonly, acute CF presents in patients who have had previous CF and who have **otherwise compromised health**. Maybe, now, there is an infection; maybe there is anemia. The initial examination helps here.

An **acute coronary syndrome,** when the person is having a heart attack due to lack of blood flow to the heart, can be a common cause of acute cardiac failure. If that patient can be taken to a coronary angiogram laboratory, the blocked artery can be opened and blood flow restored to the heart. If this occurs quickly enough, it improves the left ventricular function and makes a big difference to the person's long-term outcome.

Another cause could be an **arrhythmia**, a heart rhythm abnormality. Atrial fibrillation, particularly when the heart rate is poorly controlled and is racing, can tip a person into CF. Other fast rhythms do the same. However, the ECG results help show if this is the case.

Checking for **heart valve failure** is also important. Rupture of a valve, or acute failure of a valve, with significant flow, either way, is a major cause of cardiac distress and none of the already mentioned interventions ameliorates it. A proper diagnosis using an echo assessment followed by correction of the valve problem is this person's only chance of survival.

The last heart-related cause is *takotsubo*, or broken heart syndrome. If a person has enough emotional stress, the sympathetic nervous system can discharge so much nervous energy that it shuts down the heart.

'Takotsubo'

Takotsubo or broken heart syndrome relates to the impact emotional stress can have on the heart. This is a particular situation in which stress gives rise to severe, crushing chest pain; an experience that is hard to distinguish from a blocked artery causing a heart attack. Sufferers generally present to a hospital where they are checked for a possible problem with the coronary arteries.

Most commonly, the condition affects middle-aged women, particularly after menopause. More than 90 percent of reported cases are in women aged 58-75 years old. It can affect men, although far less frequently. Most people recover with no long-term heart damage. About 70 percent of people who present with the condition have suffered significant emotional stress. It may have been a fight, distressing circumstances in someone's life, while preparing for surgery if the person is particularly worried, or even at a football game where there is a lot of emotion.

The syndrome is hard to differentiate from a heart attack as patients have changes on their ECG that look like a heart attack and they also have raised troponin levels, detected by a blood test. However, they have not suffered a 'true' heart attack. What has happened is that after a significant outpouring of nervous activity, hormones produced from the adrenal glands impact the working of the heart muscle, suddenly weakening it. This affects the left ventricle, and so affects the pumping ability of the heart. Importantly, the diagnosis is one of exclusion as the condition has the features of a heart attack without the blocked arteries.

While the precise cause is not known, experts believe that surging stress hormones such as adrenaline can 'stun' the heart, triggering changes in heart muscle cells and coronary blood vessels that prevent the left ventricle from contracting efficiently.

The name, *takotsubo* cardiomyopathy, is taken from the Japanese word for octopus pot, a descriptive term for what the heart looks like when the condition occurs. A Japanese octopus pot has a ring at the top and a

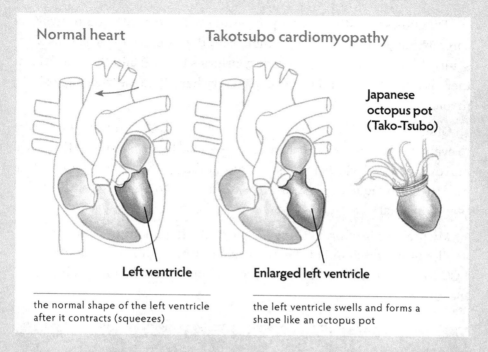

Normal heart

Takotsubo cardiomyopathy

Japanese octopus pot (Tako-Tsubo)

Left ventricle

Enlarged left ventricle

the normal shape of the left ventricle after it contracts (squeezes)

the left ventricle swells and forms a shape like an octopus pot

bulbous bottom where the body of the octopus sits. A *takotsubo* heart is characterized by the proximal parts (near the center) of the heart working, but the distal part of the left ventricle blowing out like a balloon. Instead of the heart being bullet-shaped, it becomes a collar with a bulb. **This shape is the diagnostic characteristic.** One would expect that if it were coronary artery disease, the problem would be localized to the area that is supported or supplied by the single problem coronary artery.

The condition is not that rare, occurring in probably 5-10 percent of people presenting with what appears to be a heart attack. Fortunately, it is quite uncommon for this condition to kill the person. While most of these patients recover, it can take several months. Failure to recover would prompt looking for another diagnosis. About 10 percent of patients have a second episode.

Therapies used when the heart is not pumping correctly form the basis of treatment. Because the apex of the heart balloons out and does not contract properly, it is treated as if it were a component of cardiac failure. The use of beta-blockers dampens some of the autonomic nervous system, the outpouring of the nervous system that probably caused the problem.

Diagnosis is critical. Most presenting patients undergo an invasive coronary angiogram, in which a tube, placed inside the arteries, is used to squirt dye directly into the coronary arteries to ascertain their health. If there is a narrowing or a blockage, it's very hard to make the diagnosis of *takotsubo*.

Often, instead of the invasive angiography, I use a CT coronary angiogram to evaluate the arteries. This imaging allows me to see not only if there is a narrowing or a blockage but also to look at the health of the artery, just in case there is plaque in those artery walls that could be a later problem for that individual.

My practice is to bring these people back after about three months for a follow-up ultrasound of the heart to confirm recovery and a follow-up ECG to provide a documented baseline should there be any problems in the future.

IMPORTANT POINTS

'Takotsubo' syndrome, apical-ballooning syndrome, broken heart syndrome:

- is closely linked with intense emotion
- occurs particularly in middle-aged women
- rarely causes death
- is diagnosed by exclusion, as it looks very much like a 'heart attack'
- represents up to 10 percent of people presenting with symptoms of a heart attack
- can be treated, leading to recovery in several months, with follow-up to confirm recovery recommended
- advice – don't get too emotional!

other possibilities

Once heart-related options have been excluded as the cause of the person's distress, other possibilities include infection, anemia, renal failure and pulmonary embolism. **Renal failure** leads to the retention of fluid and can overload the heart. **Pulmonary embolism** (PE) can present with features similar to acute CF. However, the cardiac failure-like features of PE affect the right-hand side of the heart. The embolism, or clot, becomes caught in the lungs and it is the right-hand side of the heart that is trying to pump the blood past the blockage. The left-hand side of the heart, which receives blood from the lungs, is not under much pressure. Still, the patient can be very ill, and it is a life-threatening condition.

IMPORTANT POINTS

Acute cardiac failure is a very serious condition. Cardiogenic shock is its extreme end.

As much as possible is being done at the same time:

- thorough examination and history
- tests and start of therapy as soon as possible
  - deploy oxygen, opiates
  - take bloods
  - provide diuretic therapy
  - ventilatory intervention
  - mechanical circulatory support (if available).

THE HEART

LIVING WITH CARDIAC FAILURE

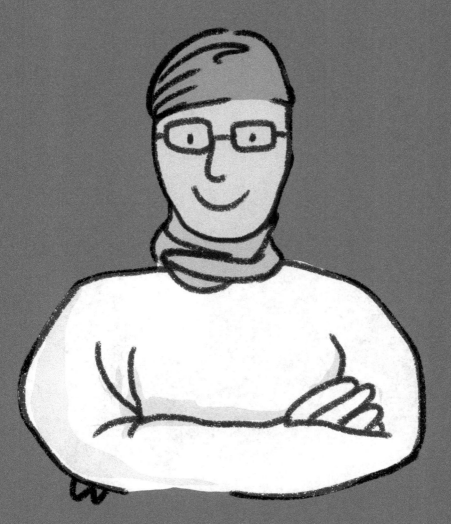

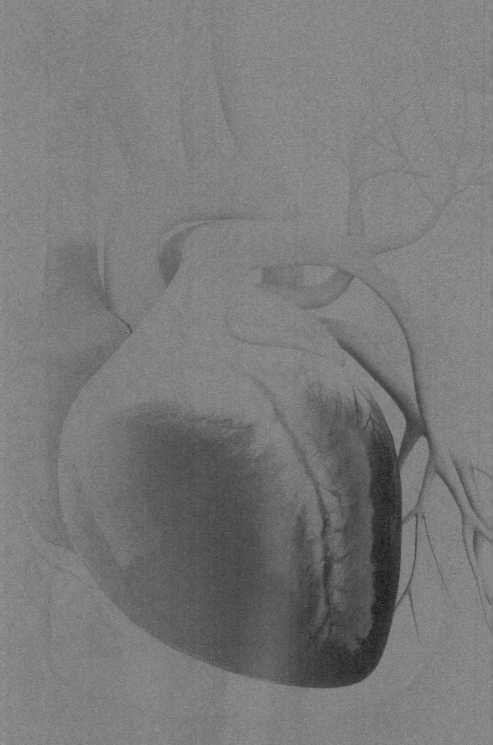

chapter 18
MANAGEMENT OF CARDIAC FAILURE – A HOLISTIC APPROACH

Cardiac failure patients are often medically complex patients. As cardiac failure becomes more prevalent with age, the patients can be older, and as people age, unfortunately, they suffer from more health issues. When a person has one or more serious conditions in addition to the primary problem, these concurrent conditions are called **co-morbidities**. As we know, common partners with CF include diabetes, renal impairment, treatment of and recovery from cancers and sometimes lung disease.

patient management

As these patients have multiple needs, they must have a good, ongoing, and regular relationship with a **trusted general practitioner** or primary care clinician. This medical practitioner becomes a fixed, connecting point in ongoing care and works closely with the various specialists who are looking after specific problems. From a heart perspective, central to this is the **cardiologist** who has experience and expertise in the management of cardiac failure and can ensure that the very best therapy is in place for the individual patient. Supporting the cardiologist are **nurse practitioners** who help implement therapies ensuring the patient has a sound understanding of the explanations and medications and making sure that there is also suitable follow-up after cardiology consultations.

What has developed over time is the understanding that, with the complexity of cardiac failure, there can be real benefits from creating **specialized units** dedicated to the care of patients with cardiac failure. **Multidisciplinary teams** staff such units. Often, these units are located in large clinics because the teams need substantial infrastructure to support them. Team members can monitor issues such as medications, blood pressure and weight as well as any devices in the unit and/or remotely and provide phone support.

Good research evidence supports the use of **nurse-led titration clinics**. Here, the patients with cardiac failure are seen by nurses who review the medication, checking that the patients are on the appropriate therapies and receiving the correct doses. For most cardiac failure medications – the ACE inhibitors, the angiotensin receptor blockers, the beta-blockers and even the neprilysin inhibitors – the highest dose possible gives patients their best benefits. Ongoing reviews and frequent checking are of the utmost importance.

Initially, I bring patients back on a regular and frequent basis so that I might holistically try to address each of the patient's issues as quickly as possible. As the patient stabilizes, as medications are uptitrated and as the patient gains a better understanding of the caring process, I then start to extend the length of time between visits. The frequency of visits can extend to 12 months once the patient has stabilized on maximally tolerated doses of appropriate therapies.

self-management

An individual's self-management and engagement are essential to ongoing care. **Self-management, paired with understanding and education, leads to ownership** of the condition. The better a patient can understand what is happening, the better the patient can understand the role of medications and why they are needed, the importance of follow-up, diet and exercise, then the better the outcome for that patient.

Remember Mary from the introduction to this book? Having been well educated about the accumulation of fluid leading to the swelling in her ankles and the development of shortness of breath, she controlled her own intervention, leading to an excellent outcome for her ongoing well-being. Not only did I educate Mary, I also included her daughters as part of Mary's management team, and it worked well for all concerned.

CAM'S JOURNEY

youthful adjustment

Not long after my 31st birthday in May 2017, I was at work grabbing a coffee when I felt light-headed and dizzy. During the previous couple of days, I'd had some weird chest pain that I thought was reflux and a left arm that felt like it had been punched. It then dawned on me that maybe these symptoms were related. I took 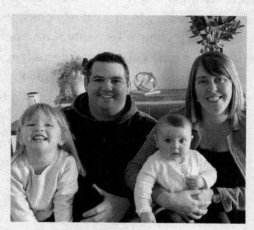 myself to the emergency department, and after a few days, and multiple tests, my diagnosis was dilated cardiomyopathy.

At first, I didn't know exactly what my diagnosis meant. Initially, I was more relieved to get out of the hospital and back home. At home, the extent of my condition started to sink in. Especially after searching Google and reading a few articles, I realized that my illness was much more serious than I had first thought. It took a good week to get my head around what I was dealing with and what lifestyle changes I needed to make. With my first daughter only nine months old, I figured I had no choice other than to make the changes.

> *It is very important not to take all that Google says at face value. Always consult your cardiologist if you have any concerns.*

The biggest challenge I had early on was with my medication. I felt like a truck had hit me. I went from being an energetic and social 31-year-old to feeling sick. I had no energy and suffered like I was battling a severe hangover 24/7. Eventually, I was able to function relatively normally.

219

However, some days were certainly harder than others.

Another truly challenging obstacle I had to come to terms with was work. Running my own business and dealing with a dozen or so employees has its stresses. In those early days, with minimal energy, there wasn't much motivation to keep things on track. My business suffered during the first few months, and that affected my mental state. Some days I felt as though my life was all doom and gloom. Eventually, I was able to overcome this as I started to come to terms with the fact that some things you can't change and there are plenty of people out there far worse off than me.

Now, thankfully, my business provides me with the freedom and lifestyle I need to deal with my day to day challenges and my growing family. Regular doctors' appointments, tests, and medications have become a normal part of my life. Importantly, my body has adapted to the side-effects of the drugs.

My friends and family have been there throughout my journey. It certainly has become much easier to deal with as time has gone by. I'm now enjoying a relatively normal life. I've learned to live with its few restraints. ♥

IMPORTANT POINTS

- CF patients often are medically complex patients.
- Patients need a good, ongoing relationship with a primary care clinician, cardiologist and supporting nurse practitioners.
- Good self-management, understanding and education lead to ownership and far better outcomes.

Lifestyle changes are an important part of cardiac failure management. A holistic approach benefits the ongoing well-being and prognosis of the patient.

chapter 19
LIFESTYLE

As well as the availability of the various drug therapies, devices and surgical options that have been outlined, **non-pharmacological management** of cardiac failure is central to care and treatment. This refers to interventions that are related to the lifestyle of the patient, which help provide more holistic care of the individual.

Non-pharmacological management complements any pharmacological management with both equally aiming to improve the patient's survival and quality of life.

fluid

Current literature supports the notion that patients who are **congested**, and have more fluid in their system than is necessary, benefit from a restricted fluid allowance per day, of about 1.5 liters. These fluid-overloaded patients exhibit symptoms such as swollen legs, a 'wet' chest, shortness of breath and a pulse in the neck that shows that the fluid pressures in the right atrium are high.

The result of limiting fluid intake for all cardiac failure patients is not clear. There are suggestions that harm could be done, with a detrimental impact on blood pressure and the kidneys as the most likely result. This is particularly so for patients who have a normal volume of bodily fluid (euvolemic) or those whose volume is slightly under (hypovolemic). Fluid intake should be discussed with your cardiologist.

salt

The National Heart Foundation of Australia recommends less than two grams of salt per day. The American Heart Association recommendation is in keeping with this – for (New York Heart Association Functional Classification of Heart Failure) Class I and II HF, less that 1.5 g/day, and because of the limited evidence from trial data, less than 3 g/day for Class III and IV HF. *(refer to the classification table on page 102)*

The body's response when it feels that the heart is not working properly is to reabsorb sodium and retain water, which is not what we want in CF. Furthermore, since certain heart medications act on the body's salt balance systems, perhaps even more caution, and, therefore, even less salt could be a good thing.

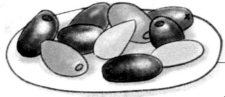

a serve of potato chips is approximately 0.16–0.19g, while 10 olives in brine will be close to 2g

exercise

There is no doubt that exercise for patients with CF is beneficial. Exercise recommendations encompass both endurance training (such as walking) and strength training (including weights). According to the current data, a combination of both produces the optimal outcome.

An individual could consult with an exercise physiologist or even a personal trainer to achieve the best results. Even without that, though, research tells us endurance training allows people to walk further with fewer symptoms, leading to an increase in general well-being. With cardiac failure linked to older age, which is allied with frailty, some strength exercises would be valuable as an aid to maintaining mobility and independence.

---

right: This is a letter I received from a patient who worked out an exercise regime for himself that proved to be highly beneficial in decreasing fluid retention and improving breathing and mobility. The good news is that the exercise will not damage his heart nor wear out his 'pig valve'. While his exercise capacity is improving or stable, there is little concern from me.

17 October, 2019

Dr. W. Bishop
Calvary Hospital
Augusta Road
LENAH VALLEY TAS 7008

Dear Warwick (sic)

I need some advice from you on a venture I started to improve my situation. We have just returned from a 24 day cruise which had an elaborate gymnasium. I availed myself of the opportunity to use the treadmill.

... my wife did 30 minutes at a time and my effort was 3 x 5 minutes with rest as required in between. It has improved my breathing and walking but most encouragingly it eliminated the big wads of phlegm I usually bring up due to water in my lungs.

I found I had to walk at 4 km/hr to allow me to do 4 steps breathing in and 4 steps breathing out to stabilize my heart rate at 120 to 130 b.p.m. so as the treadmill can be controlled and stopped instantly when required. It has helped my walking, breathing and water retention. I just wonder what the effect is on my heart and 'pig valve'. Could you please give me advice on what to monitor or watch out for. (sic)

I'm hoping to keep this up 2 to 3 times a week with your approval.

Thank you ...

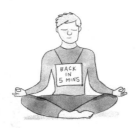

yoga

As there is no doubt that exercise is beneficial, where does yoga fit in, or does it? Its long history links physical, mental and spiritual wellbeing, and it is emerging as a prominent component in holistic medical care. Yoga therapy research links improved cardiovascular and quality of life outcomes for heart failure patients due to improvements in muscle strength, endurance and flexibility, and decreased anxiety.[18]

Many studies support the contention that yoga lowers blood pressure. This is because of the interplay between yoga and the parasympathetic nervous system (PSNS, 'rest and digest')/sympathetic (SNS, 'fight or flight') nervous system in which muscular stretch releases stress, altering the autonomic tone of the body. The sympathetic drive decreases, the blood vessels dilate, and blood pressure reduces. Studies have also shown a decrease in inflammatory markers, weight and depression. One study[19] went even further and took patients with reduced ejection fraction cardiac failure, put them through yoga, or not, for six months, and then re-evaluated their hearts. A clear benefit — a significant improvement in heart function — was shown in the group that undertook yoga.

I'm guessing they improved flexibility and, perhaps, exercise tolerance as well. Good!

Studies have also shown that yoga can decrease the recurrence of atrial fibrillation. Researchers in a University of Kansas Hospital study[20] followed a group of patients for three months as a baseline and then started a twice-weekly yoga regime with home practice. Comparing the before and after figures, yoga reduced the rates of AF by nearly 40 percent.

So, yoga is not just good for the soul, it is good for your heart. However, its use comes with the caution for CF patients to avoid rigorous or continuous-flow style yoga, classes conducted in a heated room and any breath-holding. [21] Furthermore, yoga should always be practised with care, and to the ability of the patient. Such caution will avoid any over-stretching that could result in damage to muscles and ligaments.

Isn't that fantastic? And, unbelievably, yoga can reduce the frequency of discharge of shock from implantable defibrillators.

supplements

Often, patients want to know what they can do to improve their health beyond their prescribed medication. I'm very supportive of them. Some want to make lifestyle changes and are interested in supplementation. While there is not much evidence to support the use of supplements being beneficial, there are a couple of possibilities worth considering.

fish oil

Fish oils are discussed, regularly, not only in the popular press but also in our medical literature and at meetings. Sometimes, these supplements seem to be good for the patient; sometimes, they are not so good. Sometimes, we see positive effects; sometimes, there seems to be no effect. And thanks to 'sound bite' reporting in the media, I think many people are confused.

In the past year or so several important fish oil-related trials have been undertaken. Here, I focus on one aspect and that is the scenario of cardiac failure and heart attacks; a situation in which people have experienced a heart attack that damaged the muscle and left them with CF. These people are at significantly increased risk of another heart attack. Another heart attack in an already damaged heart is **terrible news.**

In looking to the positive to help reduce further events, some data suggest that generous doses of a refined component of fish oil can reduce the risk of a recurrent heart attack in individuals

- who have established coronary artery disease,
- with high triglyceride levels, and
- who are at high risk of another event.

The REDUCE-IT trial (Reduction of Cardiovascular Events with EPA-Intervention Trial)[22] produced useful data showing that high doses (+4 g/day) of a purified fish oil derivative improved outcome substantially. So, a good quality, high dose of this fish oil constituent is beneficial to people in this group.

co-enzyme Q10 or CoQ10

People often ask about CoQ10, also called 'ubiquinone' because it is ubiquitous in the body. Well, what is it? It's a co-enzyme used for metabolism and also for antioxidation. CoQ10 is an integral part of all cellular function. Importantly, it may have a cellular role as well in failing hearts. Although some data support this role, the studies have not been big enough to draw robust conclusions. However, they have given an inkling that this agent can be beneficial.

My thought is that it might be a useful add-on. I suggest that if patients can afford it, and if it fits with their philosophy, then, give it a go as there are no suggestions at this stage that it does any harm.

While we wait for more data, it's not a bad thing to try.

selenium

Selenium is a chemical element (or mineral, as in vitamin and mineral) that supports the function of several of the body's systems, including the cardiovascular system. A recent review of BIOSTAT-CHF[23], involving an international prospective cohort of more than 2500 patients, looked at selenium concentrations and found that just over 20 percent had levels less than 70 micrograms/L, which is considered deficient. These CF patients had worse symptoms, more severe signs and poorer quality of life. They were older, and more often, women. This group had a greater all-cause mortality and though no trials show replacing or supplementing with selenium improves outcomes, it should not be harmful to ensure a good balanced and varied diet with selenium-rich foods, such as Brazil nuts, tuna, pork and some dairy products.

other supplements

A small number of trials have looked at the value of other supplements such as magnesium, hawthorn, thiamine (except in thiamine vitamin B1 deficiency), vitamin C, E and D (except in specific deficiencies). No benefits for cardiac failure patients have been shown.

diet

I encourage my patients to eat a healthy, well-balanced Mediterranean-type diet with lots of varied fresh produce, and to avoid processed food wherever possible. That way, they receive a variety of nutrients, essential minerals and vitamins from natural, broadly-based sources.

IMPORTANT POINTS

Many patients and medicos take a holistic approach to treating cardiac failure. In addition to the medications and devices, key lifestyle variants include:

fluid

- patients who are congested benefit from a restricted fluid allowance per day, of about 1.5 liters

- patients who are not congested should not necessarily limit their fluid intake

salt

- the National Heart Foundation of Australia and the American Heart Association recommend less than 2 grams of salt per day (depending on medications, even less may be better)

exercise

- any exercise is significant. A combination of endurance training (walking) and strength training (weights) gives the best outcome

(continued next page)

---

yoga

- by slowing down the sympathetic nervous system, it
  - reduces stress
  - improves stretch
  - strengthens the legs
  - improves inflammatory factors within the blood
- studies also demonstrate that yoga
  - improves heart rate variability
  - improves blood pressure
  - lowers heart rate
  - provides better sleep
  - improves quality of life

supplements

- can play a role for some patients
  - who can pay for them
  - for whom they fit, philosophically
- fish oil, CoQ10 and selenium could be worth considering
  - in most circumstances, they should not cause harm, but always use in consultation with your medical advisors

diet

- in all cases, eat a healthy, varied, fresh produce-rich diet.

[18]   *Yoga for Heart Failure: A Review and Future Research, International Journal of Yoga; 2018 May-August; 11(2): 91-98*

[19]   *A Randomized Controlled Trial to Study the Effect of Yoga Therapy on Cardiac Function and N Terminal Pro BNP in Heart Failure; Integr Med Insights. 2014; 9: 1–6; Published online 2014 Apr 1. doi: 10.4137/IMI.S13939; PMCID: PMC3981569 PMID: 24737932*

[20]   *University of Kansas Hospital (the impact of yoga on AF trial) Journal of the American College of Cardiology 2013 Mar 19; 61 (11): 1177-82*

[21]   *op. cit. Yoga for Heart Failure*

[22]   *REDUCE-IT (Cardiovascular Risk Reduction Icosapent Ethyl for Hypertriglyceridemia) N Engl J Med 2019; 380:11-22*

[23]   *BIOSTAT-CHF (A systems BIOlogy Study to TAilored Treatment in Chronic Heart Failure) European Commission CORDIS (final report summary) https://cordis.europa.eu/project/ id/242209/reporting*

         see also A systems BIOlogy Study to TAilored Treatment in Chronic Heart Failure: rationale, design, and baseline characteristics of BIOSTAT-CHF https://www.ncbi.nlm.nih.gov/ pubmed/27126231

Women and cardiac failure

chapter 20
WOMEN

Historically, cardiac failure trials have recruited men more often than women, in a ratio of about seven to three. While research has been done predominantly on men, between 40 and 50 percent of all patients with cardiac failure are women. Cardiac failure affects one to two percent of the population. That percentage increases significantly as people 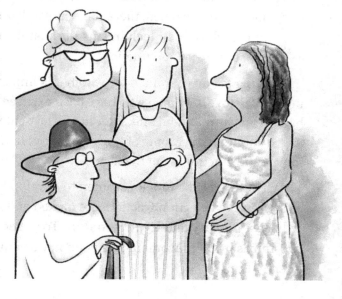 (especially men) reach 60 years of age or above, and it increases even more (especially in women) around 85 years of age or above.

Men and women have slightly different types of cardiac failure. As we know, there are two major classification characteristics of CF, reduced ejection fraction (HFrEF) and preserved ejection fraction (HFpEF). In the first, **reduced ejection fraction**, the heart does not pump properly because the pumping mechanism is not doing its job correctly. Generally, the heart looks big, is dilated, and doesn't contract well. In the second, **preserved ejection fraction,** the heart is stiff and does not relax properly. This inability of the left ventricle to relax leads to the failure of the heart as a pump, although the heart is of normal size and, surprisingly, looks as if it is pumping as it should.

Women represent a higher proportion of **preserved** ejection fraction

(HFpEF) cardiac failure sufferers. Theories for this include:

- that as women have smaller hearts than men, they could be more prone to inadequate relaxation of the heart, or diastolic dysfunction;

- that women may be more prone to microvascular disease, a disease of the very, very small arteries that supply the heart muscle, and

- that as there is a notably higher incidence of HFpEF in post-menopausal women, there could be a link between hormonal changes and underlying mechanisms of diastolic function, which lead to preserved ejection fraction.

Another group of women for whom it is important to be aware of their medical history is women who have been exposed to chemotherapy during breast cancer treatment and, later in life, present with shortness of breath. As we know already, some of the agents used in treating breast cancer can impact the functioning of the heart.

When the risk factors for women to develop heart failure, particularly with preserved ejection fraction, are looked at, there are two outstanding red flags: **obesity** and **hypertension**. Together they contribute to about two-thirds of CF in women. The good news is that both are amenable to intervention.

These are significant areas of which to be aware. Potential problems should be targeted and dealt with appropriately earlier in life.

Another risk factor is **diabetes**. Diabetes is an independent risk factor for the development of CF. Patients with diabetes are at increased risk of coronary artery disease, and therefore, cardiac failure, if a lack of blood flow damages the heart. Their raised glucose levels also alter the metabolic function of the heart muscle. Raised sugars and insulin, too, are linked to activation of the sympathetic nervous system, increased inflammation and increased fibrosis, all less than desirable for looking after your heart.

Heart failure with preserved ejection fraction can often be overlooked in women. Both women and men sufferers present with one or more of the three classic symptoms, shortness of breath, swollen legs, fatigue. However, it appears that **depression** is more common in women and they often experience a **worse quality of life**.

If cardiac failure is not front-of-mind for a primary care practitioner, CF symptoms can be misdiagnosed. For example, wheezing, coughing, and shortness of breath can be misinterpreted as worsening symptoms of chronic obstructive pulmonary disease or even asthma when it could be CF. Tricky!

challenging to treat

HFpEF can be challenging to treat. Lowering elevated blood pressure is an important starting point, and some diuretic therapy might help with symptoms. There is not much research giving insight into interventions that may improve mortality in the longer term for this group. This lack of research places substantial significance on identifying and implementing **early** prevention strategies.

The European Society of Cardiology meeting held in Paris, August-September 2019, looked at the results of the PARAGON-HF trial. This trial studied heart failure with preserved ejection fraction in people who have all the symptoms of heart failure, including brain natriuretic peptide elevation, but an ejection fraction of greater than 45 percent. The hope was that the PARAGON-HF trial[24] would show that entresto – a combination of an AT2 receptor blocker, valsartan, and a neprilysin inhibitor, sacubitril – would help patients with preserved ejection fraction heart failure.

The trial showed a small reduction in the death rate and a small reduction in total hospital events but no clinically significant data pointed to benefits from entresto over valsartan used alone. That the neprilysin inhibitor and the AT2 receptor blocker combination did not show statistical significance in improving outcomes for patients with preserved ejection fraction was disappointing because currently there is no other intervention to help this group of, mainly, women. Although there was subgroups analysis within that trial that suggested women and patients with lower ejection fractions did better on entresto, neither was statistically significant. As a result, current heart failure management did not change. Heart failure with preserved ejection fraction is a treatment space with few answers. It is an area that needs further research and development.

[24]   (The New England Journal of Medicine, 24 October 2019)   https://www.nejm.org/doi/full/10.1056/NEJMoa1908655
also
European Society of Cardiology media release
https://www.escardio.org/The-ESC/Press-Office/Press-releases/paragon-hf-misses-endpoint-in-preserved-heart-failure-but-benefit-noted-in-some-patients

CASE STUDY – JILL

shortness of breath, wheezing, enlarged heart, pulmonary effusion, HFrEF, had earlier been treated for breast cancer

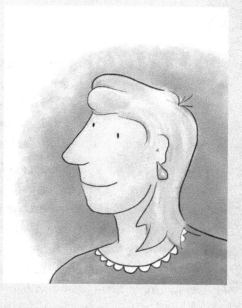

Jill, 71, was very sick when I met her at the beginning of 2019.

She was in the hospital having presented with shortness of breath, crackling and wheezing, and was being treated for pneumonia. A chest x-ray showed what could have been a lung infection. The image also showed an enlarged heart and a pulmonary effusion, meaning that there was an accumulation of fluid between the layers of tissues that line the lungs and the chest wall. Evidence of a big heart on x-ray suggested that it might not be an infection. A subsequent echocardiogram demonstrated clearly that her problem was cardiac failure. She had an ejection fraction of 25 percent. Her heart was racing. She had features of fluid overload. She was in trouble. It was at that stage that the medical team looking after her invited me to become involved.

On speaking with Jill, I learned that her health had been deteriorating progressively for 12 months, culminating in her admission to hospital. Significantly, about 18 months earlier, she had been diagnosed with cancer of the breast. She had had surgery and chemotherapy. Exposure to the chemotherapeutic agents used in breast cancer treatment might have caused Jill's heart function to lessen.

I started Jill on standard therapy for cardiac failure. I put her on an ACE inhibitor, a beta-blocker, and, because of clear features of fluid

overload, I also prescribed a diuretic. Jill was apprehensive about taking medications, especially as they would lower her blood pressure, which had been always recorded as 'low' over the years.

The ACE inhibitors lower blood pressure; the beta-blockers can lower blood pressure as well and slow down the heart, and the diuretics will also lower blood pressure.

I explained to her the crucial need to reduce the amount of fluid in her body, adding that once that occurred, she would experience a benefit from her heart needing to do less work since the volume of fluid in her body would have decreased. By educating her and engaging her in that discussion, she was happy to take those medications.

I saw her in my rooms two weeks later. A follow-up x-ray showed, quite pleasingly, that the pleural effusions had resolved, so the fluid that had been within the chest cavity had cleared. The body had reabsorbed it, and the diuretics had expelled it via the kidneys. Looking at her legs for swelling and at her neck for the jugular venous pressure, she was clearly much nearer to a healthy fluid balance than when I first saw her. Her heart rate had come down from over 100 beats per minute to nearer 85 b.p.m; not exactly where we wanted it to be but certainly a significant improvement.

At that appointment, I started to up-titrate the agents that I had started Jill on while she was in the hospital. This is standard guideline management. I started to gently increase the ACE inhibitor, ramipril, and the beta-blocker, which was bisoprolol. I also gave Jill guidelines on how to use the fluid tablet, furosemide, on an as-needed basis when she noticed a return of either shortness of breath or swelling of ankles.

I saw her several times, in relatively quick succession to ensure she continued to progress well while checking renal function, blood pressure and her toleration to the drugs. Over the course of these visits, we up-titrated her medications to attain a maximum therapeutic advantage. She did well.

After about three months, we did another echocardiogram to re-evaluate her heart function. The results showed that her ejection fraction had increased from 25 percent to between 40 and 45 percent. This was a really good outcome. Her health had improved substantially. She was tolerating the tablets. She felt much better. We were both happy with the result.

Nine months later (about the time of writing this book), Jill remains stable and well on her therapies. As we know from recent literature, she needs to remain on those medications for the remainder of her life. However, Jill, fortunately, is doing well, and there has been a significant recovery in her cardiac function.

Jill's progress is a pleasing outcome for all.

IMPORTANT POINTS

Women

- account for between 40 and 50 percent of all cases of heart failure
    - that percentage increases, especially in women older than 85 years
- are more likely than men to have heart failure with preserved ejection fraction (HFpEF)
    - which can be difficult to diagnose
    - which can be difficult to treat
    - with blood pressure and obesity as significant risk factors (these should be targeted early in life)
- with a history of chemotherapy treatment for breast cancer may present with shortness of breath later in life, which could possibly indicate CF.

Living with cardiac failure raises many questions and uncertainties. Answers to some common and interesting queries are next.

chapter 21
DOCTOR, CAN I ...?

The diagnosis of any illness raises questions for patients and their family, carers and friends. As we have seen, the symptoms of cardiac failure can improve for some patients, in many cases giving them back a zest for life. Following are some of the most commonly asked questions.

drive

With the diagnosis of cardiac failure, it is prudent to check the health guidelines for the state, county or country in which you live if you want to continue to drive. If your condition is stable and well-controlled, then a private vehicle driver's license is generally permitted.

If a person requires a driver's license for a commercial vehicle, such as a bus, truck, taxi, then specific requirements apply. The particular circumstance of a person having an implantable cardiac defibrillator that restarts the heart rules out most people from driving a commercial vehicle. However, the regulations are worthwhile working through as you may be able to obtain a conditional license.

So, for both types of licenses, please check the regulations in your local jurisdiction. In general, however, CF should not stop you from driving. The best and safest option is to go through the local guidelines with your cardiologist.

One of the repercussions of driving, if legally you should **not** be driving, is that if you were to be involved in an accident, it could have severe consequences for any insurance claim. Another, of course, is having an accident and severely injuring yourself and others.

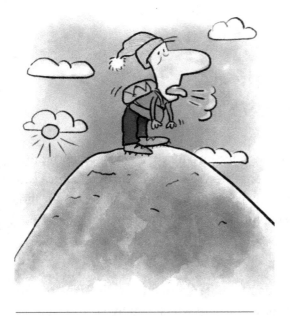

travel

The simple answer to the question, "Can I travel?" is, "Yes, possibly." The "possibly" means that you need to be aware of your destination and traveling conditions. For any patients whose condition is unstable, air travel is **not** a good idea.

The altitude of your destination and decompression in an aircraft cabin are serious considerations.

If you have cardiac failure, doing the Annapurna Circuit or an Everest Base camp trek should probably not be on your travel list.

As a traveler, you need to think about your arrival destination. Flying to a high-altitude destination could precipitate problems because of changes in oxygenation. Flying from sea level directly to a high-altitude destination such as Las Pas, in Bolivia, could cause acute decompensation and, certainly, decreased exercise capacity.

Decompression in the cabin of an aircraft, to an altitude of between 8000 and 10,000 feet, is something that you need to factor into your decision-making. Less oxygen than you are used to at sea level could destabilize or worsen your condition. Generally, that change in oxygenation should not be a problem on short trips for patients who are taking their medications, have been recently reviewed, and whose condition has stabilized and is well maintained.

Longer trips present complications.

Even for people without cardiac failure, long trips are hard work.

The timing of medications is important, both on the ground and in the air. Fluid tablets, for example, could pose challenges including those brought about by the availability of, and access to, toilets. Dehydration can easily occur on a long-haul flight, or you might become cramped and, due to lack of movement, run the risk of clots forming in the legs. Deep vein thrombosis

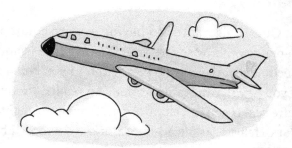

(DVT) is concerning because the clot can break off and make its way to the lungs. The resulting pulmonary embolism (PE) is a very serious – potentially life-threatening – condition. So, thinking of undertaking a long-haul flight is something that needs thoughtful consideration.

How does a traveler balance fluid retention and the need for hydration, especially on a long-haul flight? Can alcohol be consumed safely? How often should a person move or stretch? Can medication, such as low-dose anticoagulation drugs, be prescribed to prevent blood clots? Travel possibilities would make a great conversation with your cardiologist.

have vaccinations

Vaccinations are vital. With cardiac failure, you are at increased risk of contracting multiple, different conditions. Work with your doctor to ensure that you are appropriately vaccinated.

Pneumococcal, COVID-19 and influenza vaccines are highly recommended if you have impaired heart function. No argument!

have sex

Questions related to having sex are common. The bottom line is, it depends on how severe your heart failure is and your ability to exercise. Technically, there is no restriction to you being physically active sexually if you have cardiac impairment. In reality, though, you need the energy to have sex. If you can climb several, say three, flights of stairs and have a New York Heart Classification of 1 or 2, you should have the exercise capacity required for sexual intimacy.

Some cardiac failure medications can lead to erectile dysfunction. Drugs, such as spironolactone, can have a feminizing effect, and beta-blockers can dampen sexual function.

This leads to the question, "Can I use Viagra?" Generally, the Viagra-type, phosphodiesterase inhibitor drugs can be used. However, there is a cautionary note. If coronary artery disease (narrowed arteries) caused your heart failure, then be very careful to check you are not taking nitrate-based medication which includes the spray under the tongue. These medications dilate blood vessels to help the arteries. They react with Viagra and can drop the blood pressure profoundly and dangerously. It would be wise to have a conversation with your cardiologist or your local doctor.

stop taking the tablets

That some people recover from their cardiac failure poses the question, "Can those who have recovered stop taking their medication?" Very recently, the TRED HF study[25] looked for the first time at what would happen in people who had had cardiac failure, had been given appropriate medications, their heart function had recovered, and then medications were withdrawn. This randomized trial over several years demonstrated a 30 percent recurrence rate for those who had stopped their medication.

Sorry! But that's the best way to look after you in the long term.

One-in-three is too high a risk, too high a gamble with the patient's future, so the recommendation is that if you have cardiac failure, you are on medication for the remainder of your life.

get better

There is no straightforward answer to the question, "Can I get better?" When I went to medical school many years ago, we used to say that about a third of CF patients got better, a third got worse and about a third stayed the same. That was in the time before the development of ACE inhibitors and other, more recent, medications, and before the current understanding of the place of the neurohumoral response, hormones and the autonomic nervous system in CF. It was also before the invention of some of the remarkable devices we now have available for use in treatment.

Observation within my practice indicates that with these fantastic new therapies, many more people improve and many other people remain stable. Today, it is far less common to see people deteriorate.

Unfortunately, for the individual, there is no crystal ball and only time will tell. This makes it imperative for patients to adhere to their treatment plan and have follow-up consultations.

DOC, WHAT ABOUT ...?

frequency of consultations

Patients want to know how often they should see their doctor. This answer is simple. It depends on the **stability** of your cardiac failure.

After a new diagnosis of CF stabilizes in the hospital and the person is discharged, I then monitor that person closely through visits to my rooms. Initially, visits are weekly, for a week or two, to ensure the fluid balance and kidney function are good; then, the span stretches out to fortnightly and monthly. When patients have had their medications adjusted appropriately, have maintained renal function, feel well and are functioning as well as possible then often I'm happy to see them annually.

It is important that patients know they do not need to wait until the annual check-up to see me. If they have worries or questions, an appointment can be made for any time, and the sooner the better.

Bloods need to be checked regularly, especially in the early stages, to ensure that fluid volume, medications and kidney function are balanced. Electrocardiograms (ECGs) assess the heart rate at rest, and these results may alter the medications. Further echos are also taken. Often, the at-presentation poor-function result may show improvement at three months, and so it is likely to be repeated at six months. It is not uncommon for stable patients with a history of cardiac failure to have their heart scanned with ultrasound every year, or two.

pregnancy

Cardiac failure and pregnancy present a **complicated** and **specialist area**.

A woman, born with congenital cardiac abnormalities, may live to an age at which she wants to have children. This is an intricate situation; one that is dealt with by an adult congenital heart specialist, as the differences in congenital heart disease can be substantial.

Some women can have dilated cardiomyopathy as the result of an infection, or as an inherited condition. Close collaboration with your doctor is essential, as the degree of the problem with the heart can be a significant factor in making appropriate plans.

The very process of being pregnant can lead to a very rare condition called dilated cardiomyopathy of pregnancy. While it seems to resolve itself on delivery, the baby might be delivered early to help the mother. As it can recur with future pregnancies, a conversation with your specialist about risk is highly recommended.

Another important conversation arises if either parent has a family history of an inherited cardiac condition. The risk of transmission and the consequences for the child and the family should be discussed with a geneticist or other knowledgeable specialist.

Being aware of these situations and planning a pregnancy is more valuable than being surprised and reactive. In order to avoid any unplanned or dangerous pregnancies, contraception becomes very important. From a practical perspective, a vasectomy for the man is the best contraception for the woman. A low-dose pill carries a small risk of increased risk of clot formation, while barrier methods are not the most effective form of contraception and should be used carefully.

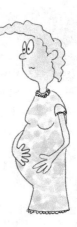

the weather

While talking about the weather often arises as a complaint, the weather, in relation to cardiac failure, is a healthy topic. Be aware:

- that marked changes in temperature, particularly hot days, can be detrimental to the body's fluid balance, as the arteries and the capillaries open up and swelling occurs;

- of your fluid intake;

- of your fluid output, and

- of the physical effort you may make on hot days.

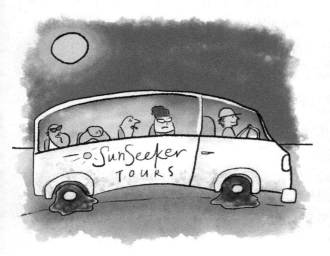

Our CF tourists! When I was in Darwin, in the Northern Territory, many years ago, we used to wait for the southerners to come north and suffer CF as the hotter temperatures significantly altered their autonomic nervous system. The visitors changed their fluid intake and lost different amounts of sweat through either respiration or perspiration. This really 'threw a spanner in the works' by bringing on swollen legs, oedema, shortness of breath. The situation was not helped if they were traveling on a tourist coach and not wanting to take diuretics!

coffee

One or two coffees for people with heart failure are okay, and may even be beneficial. After all, a cup of satisfying coffee puts a smile on your face, which is not a bad thing. Three, four or five a day is getting into problem territory. Coffee is a stimulant and you do not want to be driving your heart too hard.

alcohol

Alcohol's implication in the development of cardiac failure means it is off the menu for many sufferers.

If your heart function is:

- **low** – alcohol can be a toxin;

- **not too bad** – and a glass of wine is important to you, then please speak with your cardiologist. With clear guidelines for its consumption, alcohol may not be completely out of bounds. It is a case-by-case situation.

palliative care

One of my most difficult conversations involves palliative care for cardiac failure patients. Early recognition and acceptance that the journey can be a long one, and towards the end, pretty rough, is valuable. Among the benefits provided by good palliative care are:

- support for the carer,

- home supports to make life easier,

- medicine to ease
    - the challenges of breathing,
    - any anxiety around air hunger.

Care, consideration, respect, dignity and minimization of symptoms is available for the patient, and, also importantly, support exists for the carer, family, and others who are close.

Unfortunately, the conversation about palliative care is often not started early enough. Although it is a discussion no-one wants to have, I encourage cardiologists, patients and all those closely involved to begin this conversation sooner rather than later.

IMPORTANT POINTS

Can I

- **drive** – check the regulations in your local jurisdiction, and be guided by your cardiologist

- **travel** – yes, possibly, if your condition is stable

  - on all trips, be aware of cabin decompression and arrival altitude

  - on long distance flights, also be aware of timing of medication, dehydration, lack of movement

- **vaccinations** – vital; pneumococcal vaccine, especially, is highly recommended as are COVID-19 and influenza vaccines

- **have sex** – dependent on the severity of you CF and your exercise capacity

  - some medications can cause problems

  - Viagra-like medications can interact with other medications and can drop BP dangerously

- **stop taking tablets** – no

- **get better** – with today's medical and surgical interventions, the condition of many more people improves than previously was the case, even 20-30 years ago, and the condition deteriorates in fewer people. Many other people remain stable.

(continued next page)

What about

- **frequency of consultations** – this will depend on how stable the CF is and could range from weekly to annually.

- **pregnancy** – a complicated and specialist area

- **the weather** – be aware of the body's fluid balance, especially on hotter days

- **coffee** – no more than one or two cups a day as coffee is a stimulant

- **alcohol** – if your heart function is,
  - low, no, as it can be a toxin
  - not too bad, please discuss with your cardiologist

- **palliative care** – good palliative care is available. It is a discussion to have with all concerned sooner rather than later.

Discussion with your cardiologist about any of these factors, which apply to you, is very important.

---

[25]   Withdrawal of pharmacological treatment for heart failure in patients with recovered dilated cardiomyopathy (TRED-HF): an open-label, pilot, randomised trial
published: November 11, 2018
The Lancet, volume 393, issue 10166, page 61-73, January 05, 2019 https://www.thelancet.com/article/S0140-6736(18)32484-X/fulltext

An exciting future lies ahead for the evolution of cardiac failure treatment if the significant strides made during the past 40 years continue.

epilogue
BEYOND THE HORIZON

Although cardiac failure has been with us for a very long time, advances in its treatment belong exclusively to recent centuries, and it has only been in modern decades that therapies – both drug and device – have enjoyed significant evolution. Now having come to a space of excellent treatment options, the future could hold exciting, science-fiction-type opportunities for CF sufferers.

For a very long time, cardiac failure was uncommon in the community. It wasn't prevalent because people did not live long enough to develop it, and, there were other circumstances, particularly infections and injury from accidents, that caused people's death. When it was seen, it often related to nutritional deficiency, such as beriberi, a lack of thiamine caused by a very poor diet or alcoholism. This lack can give rise to cardiac failure called wet beriberi, in which vasodilation leads to swelling, and, ultimately, congestive cardiac failure. Besides nutritional deficiencies, congenital abnormalities – where patients had a structural defect of the heart that led to excessive wear and tear – developed into CF.

Specific and targeted therapies for cardiac failure began appearing around the turn of the 19th century. These were centered on mercurial agents to help diuresis, or to draw fluid from the body. Until then, the use of leeches and bloodletting were the remedies.

I'm glad (as I'm guessing you would be) we've moved on from there.

From then until the 1980-90s, the use of diuretics, digoxin and bed rest were the mainstay therapies. Gradually, though, understanding and treatment options evolved. In the 1980s, drugs to lower blood pressure, the vasodilators, came into play. Cardiac failure management strategy then centered on removing fluid using diuretics, supporting the muscle of the heart using digoxin, and reducing the heart's workload using the vasodilator agents. In the 1990s, neurohumoral agents, those agents that work in the renin-angiotensin-aldosterone system, in particular, the ACE inhibitors, were developed. This neurohumoral modulation started a new era in the management of cardiac failure, which saw it progress from dealing with mechanical issues to incorporating treatment of the environment in which the heart was failing. Developmental work in the neurohumoral space continues today, especially with agents that act within the neprilysin system. These agents, too, modify the heart's environment.

So, in our modern world, we still use the old remedies of diuretics and digoxin, and the vasodilators, even now, are prescribed from time to time. Recently, the neurohumoral management of CF has received much attention:

- renin-angiotensin-aldosterone system (RAAS) blockers, which are both angiotensin-converting enzyme (ACE) inhibitors and angiotensin II (AT2) blockers;

- beta-blockers, which alter the sympathetic nervous system;

- aldosterone blockers, which change the way the body reabsorbs sodium, and

- neprilysin inhibitors, which act on the chemical messengers involved in supporting heart function.

Our current century has also seen the introduction of implanted mechanical devices to support medical therapy for individuals with CF. These therapies include:

- cardiac defibrillators which can restart the heart should it develop a life-threatening rhythm (significant for people with cardiac failure due to bad arteries);

- cardiac resynchronization therapy, where, if there is an electrical timing issue within the heart in which the heart contractions are no longer synchronous, the device can improve synchrony;

- left ventricular assist devices (LVAD), manufactured pumps that help the heart do the work it should be doing by itself but can't because it is failing. The LVAD acts as a bridge to potential recovery or heart transplantation, and

- (emerging) calcium modulation devices which provide a signal into the heart to alter the way the heart muscle works through calcium stimulation, using electrical impulses.

- And, of course, there is the remarkable heart transplant.

This fantastic array of medicines, supported by extraordinary devices, lowers morbidity and mortality rates and improves the quality of life for many CF patients around the world.

Our modern advances are providing a much brighter future for cardiac failure sufferers, already. Enticing prospects are drawing us into the future.

what will the future bring?

As we ponder future possibilities, we know that work using **stem cells** is already underway. This novel and exciting technique involves researchers drawing out undifferentiated cells from the patient's bone marrow and introducing them into the heart, hoping that they take on the local characteristics and functions of the heart muscle cells (the myocytes) and restore function to the heart. Although much work still needs to be done, it is a very exciting and promising area.

Specific **genes** that play certain roles within the heart are also attracting research attention. If these particular genes could be altered, then improved function of the heart in the longer term might be the outcome.

Cell implantation is another field of investigation. This process means that cells, such as a person's heart cells, are grown outside of the body and then transplanted back into the individual. Science fiction? Technology is becoming available that points to this as a real possibility in the next decade or so.

Transplantation has been the focus of much investigative work in recent years. One fascinating area is **xenotransplantation,** (*xenos*, foreign) which is the process of grafting or transplanting organs, tissues or cells between different animal species.

Already, pig heart valves are used in some cases of heart valve replacement. Fortunately, in this setting, rejection is not an issue. As porcine (pig) genetic markers are surprisingly close to human beings, pig tissue is used for this technique. If new hearts for cardiac failure patients could be 'grown' from special pigs developed to match humans closely enough to avoid rejection, then a new heart may not be rejected by the recipient's body.

While we currently have some excellent therapies, coming decades are sure to take us into fascinating new areas of discovery.

All of the above, and so much of our focus, relates to treatment. And rightly so. However, as this book was very close to completion, a 'landmark' change in diagnosis was being heralded around the world. An **international consensus statement**, released publicly on 1 March, 2021, has redefined the classification and staging of heart failure into a more standardized and rational system.

The new document "Universal Definition and Classification of Heart Failure" has been developed by the Heart Failure Society of America, the Heart Failure Association of the European Society of Cardiology, and the Japanese Heart Failure Society, and has been endorsed by international professional groups. It involved the participation of 14 countries and six continents.

In the Preamble, the authors write that this document aims to provide a universal definition of HF that is "clinically relevant, simple but conceptually comprehensive". They say that the new definition is long overdue because the current system was inconsistent, depending on the basis for diagnosis. This redefinition will bring benefit not only to cardiologists but to the many other medical practitioners involved in the diagnosis, treatment and management of heart failure. *(for further detail, please see appendix 3)*

This is perhaps the perfect note on which to end our discussion on this complex condition that is currently in a state of dynamic change and exciting possibility. Wishing for this resource to help you live as well as possible for as long as possible.

Dr Warrick Bishop
Hobart, Tasmania, Australia
August 2021

APPENDIX 1

drugs of cardiac failure

class of drug	generic name	trade name
diuretic, renin/aldosterone blocker	spironolactone eplerenone spironolactone	Aldactone
diuretic, loop	furosemide	Lasix
angiotensin-converting enzyme (ACE) inhibitor	captopril enalapril ramipril perindopril	Capoten Vasotec Tritace Coversyl
angiotensin II (AT2) receptor blocker (ARB)	candesartan valsartan telmisartan	Atacand Diovan Micardis
beta-blocker	carvedilol bisoprolol metoprolol nebivolol	Dilatrend Bicor Toprol XL Bystolic
neprilysin inhibitor	sacubitril with an ARB	Entresto
hyperpolarization-activated cyclic nucleotide-gated (HCN) channel blockers	ivabradine	Coralan
cardiac glycosides	digoxin	Lanoxin
vasodilators	hydralazine	Apresoline
nitrates	isosorbide mononitrate	Monodur
sodium-glucose transport inhibitors	empaglifozin dapaglifozin	Jardiance Farxiga

action	side-effects	monitoring
sodium loss fluid loss reduces BP	raised potassium low BP feminizes males	renal function BP tolerability
increases urine production fluid loss	renal impairment low BP	dehydration renal function
lowers BP	renal impairment low BP cough	renal function BP tolerability
lowers BP	renal impairment low BP	renal function BP tolerability
slows heart lowers BP	fatigue low BP asthma	heart rate BP tolerability
lowers BP heart tonic	low BP	BP
slows heart	slow heart visual disturbance	heart rate
improves contraction	nausea rhythm disturbance	blood levels
lowers BP	lowers BP	BP
lowers BP	headache contra-indicated with Viagra-type meds	BP
glucose and sodium loss	dehydration thrush	renal function blood sugar

timelines

item	test	frequency
heart function	echocardiogram ('echo')	in acute cardiac failure, could be as often as weekly
		in chronic cardiac failure, several months after appropriate therapy in place, then yearly if 'stable'
renal function	blood electrolytes or renal function blood test	acute, could be as often as daily.
		chronic, weekly for up to months after appropriate therapy in place, then extending as 'stable'
blood pressure	measure blood pressure and check history from patient	acute, could be as often as several times daily.
		chronic, weekly for up to months after appropriate therapy in place' then extending as 'stable'
heart rate	feel pulse and also with electrocardiogram (ECG)	acute, could be continuous, then daily
		chronic, weekly for up to months after appropriate therapy in place, then extending as 'stable'
diuretics eg: furosemide	weight	daily, or in accordance with use of diuretic
	see renal function and blood pressure	weight related to use of diuretic
		see renal function and blood pressure
agents that block renin and aldosterone eg: ACE inhibitors, ARBs, spironolactone	see renal function and blood pressure	see renal function and blood pressure

item	test	frequency
beta-blockers eg: carvidilol, bisoprolol, metoprolol	see heart rate and blood pressure	see heart rate and blood pressure
neprilysin (naturetic peptide breakdown) inhibitors eg: sacubitril	see renal function and blood pressure	see renal function and blood pressure remember, do not use with ACE-inhibitors
ivabradine	see heart rate	see heart rate
mental wellbeing	depression questionnaire	on presentation, then 6-12 monthly
pacemaker	pacemaker interrogation	6-12 monthly
bi-ventricular pacemaker	pacemaker interrogation	maximum 6 monthly
defibrillator	pacemaker interrogation	maximum 6 monthly
clinical follow up	review with cardiologist	monthly to 3 monthly, initially to maximize meds maximum 12 monthly
inherited heart problems (cardiomyopathy)	genetic echo	genetic testing done once repeated echo may be required for monitoring, sometimes yearly, sometimes less frequent immediate family also checked for inheritance

Action of agents

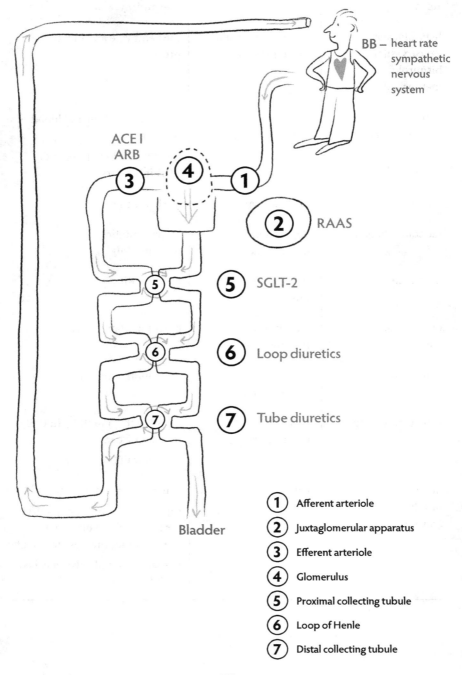

BB – heart rate
sympathetic
nervous
system

ACE I
ARB

③ ④ ①

② RAAS

⑤ SGLT-2

⑥ Loop diuretics

⑦ Tube diuretics

Bladder

① Afferent arteriole
② Juxtaglomerular apparatus
③ Efferent arteriole
④ Glomerulus
⑤ Proximal collecting tubule
⑥ Loop of Henle
⑦ Distal collecting tubule

APPENDIX 2

UNDERSTANDING THE QRS COMPLEX

As we know, there are four main chambers within the heart: a right atrium (top)- right ventricle (bottom) combination and a left atrium- left ventricle combination. Blood (deoxygenated) flows from the body into the right side of the heart. It is then pumped to the lungs for gas exchange before being returned (oxygentated) to the left side of the heart, to be pumped back around the body for use.

electrical activity in a normal heart

heartbeat starts at the top of the heart

↯

electrical impulse travels through atria

↯

atrial contraction

↯

electrical impulse passes through 'gate' to the bottom of the heart

↯

special cells act like copper wires, spreading the electrical signal through the main pumping chambers, the ventricles

↯

ventricular contraction

the electricity of the heart

It is the right atrium (top right of the heart) in which the **sinoatrial (SA) node** acts as the heart's pacemaker, setting the beat for the rest of the heart.

All the cells of the heart have an automatic depolarization system; this is called **automaticity**. This means that if you were to leave some of the cells out on a table, you could watch the cells contract as the electrical activity across the membrane changes. These cells leak sodium, potassium and calcium slowly and spontaneously until the charge across the membrane hits a threshold. When that threshold is reached, the change in the electrical potential over the membrane sets off an electrical trigger, called the action potential, which is the electrical depolarization of the cell (lots of sodium and calcium flooding into the cell). This sets off the muscle fibrils and, thereby, the contraction within those cells.

This is the 'electricity' of the heart. The cells in the sinoatrial node in the right atrium have the fastest tendency for this leakage of minerals, so they have the fastest depolarization cycle of any of the cells in the heart. That is why they set the beat.

Another fascinating thing about heart muscle cells, apart from their leaking membranes, is that they are all connected. Each cell connects to the next, to the next, to the next by special receptors between the cells that interlace and interconnect. These connections allow the electrical activity to flow rapidly through those cells. Those cells acting as one is called a **syncytium**.

When the sinoatrial node fires off, it leads to a wave of electrical activity (similar to a Mexican wave). Having started at the SA node, the wave moves from right to left through the atria. Before flowing

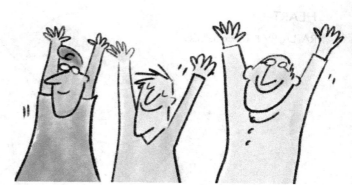

into the ventricles, the electrical activity passes through a fibrous ring that separates the atria and the ventricles. The fibrous ring does not allow the passage of electricity but has a particular point where the electrical activity can travel from the top to the bottom of the heart. This point is the **atrioventricular (AV) node.** This node acts as a gatekeeper, holding the passage of the electrical activity for about one-tenth of a second. This delay ensures the ventricles beat **after** the atria.

Helping to distribute the electrical activity from the AV node through the ventricles are more specialized cells, called Purkinje fibers, that act like copper wires. The heart contracts and then it goes back to normal, until the cells in the sinoatrial node fire up again and elicit the next contraction (heartbeat). Think of squid moving through the water: synchronous, coordinated, smooth. This is what the heart **should** do.

the electrocardiogram

An electrocardiogram (ECG) provides a non-invasive test that reads the electrical signals that activate the heart muscle and its pumping action. Twelve electrodes, which are placed at various positions on the upper torso, monitor the electrical flow, allowing the activity to be seen from different perspectives. The result is printed out or viewed on a screen.

QRS complex

The electrical activity in the atria is referred to as a **P wave,** and it reflects

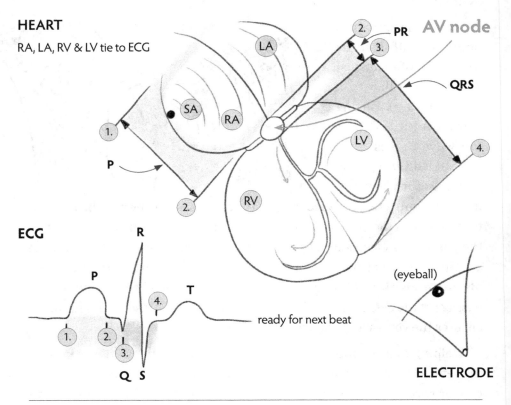

Imagine the electrode is an eyeball that sees the electrical impulse relative to the amount of current, with the current going to the electrode as an upright deflection or away, as a downward deflection. The P, Q, R, S and T waves show normal electrical flow.

atrial depolarization or the electrical flow. As the electrical impulses pass through the AV node and then on to the special distribution cells, a **QRS complex** is created, reflecting the depolarization of the major muscle of the heart. The last part of the electrical heartbeat is the **T wave,** and this is the return of normal repolarization to the heart muscle, ready for the next beat.

So, in a normal, healthy heart, sinus rhythm produces a beautiful synchronous atrial contraction followed by a beautiful synchronous ventricular contraction; a P wave, followed by a QRS complex, and a T wave.

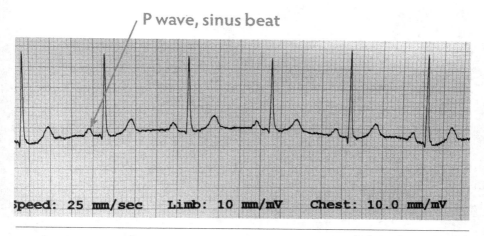

P wave, sinus beat

Speed: 25 mm/sec   Limb: 10 mm/mV   Chest: 10.0 mm/mV

sinus rhythm as shown on an ECG

APPENDIX 3

CONSENSUS STATEMENT

Universal Definition and Classification of Heart Failure: A Report of the Heart Failure Society of America, Heart Failure Association of the European Society of Cardiology, Japanese Heart Failure Society and Writing Committee of the Universal Definition of Heart Failure
Endorsed by Canadian Heart Failure Society, Heart Failure Association of India, the Cardiac Society of Australia and New Zealand, and the Chinese Heart Failure Association

Biykem BozkurtMD, PhD, Chair; Andrew JS Coats DM, DSC, Hiroyuki Tsutsui MD, co-chair; Magdy Abdelhamid MD, Stamatis Adamopoulos MD, Nancy Albert PhD, CCNS, CHFN, CCRN, NE-BC ,Stefan D. Anker MD, PhD, John Atherton MBBS, PhD, Michael Böhm MD, Javed Butler MD, MPH, MBA, Mark H. Drazner MD, MSc, G. Michael Felker MD, MHS, Gerasimos Filippatos MD, Gregg C. Fonarow MD, Mona Fiuzat PharmD, Juan-Esteban Gomez-Mesa MD, Paul Heidenreich MD, Teruhiko Imamura MD, PhD, James Januzzi MD, Ewa A. Jankowska MD, PhD, Prateeti Khazanie MD, MPH, Koichiro Kinugawa MD, PhD, Carolyn S.P. Lam, MBBS, FRCP, PhD, Yuya Matsue MD, PhD, Marco Metra MD, Tomohito Ohtani MD, PhD, Massimo Francesco Piepoli MD, PhD, Piotr Ponikowski MD, PhD, Giuseppe M.C. Rosano MD, PhD, Yasushi Sakata MD, PhD, Petar Seferović MD, PhD, Randall C. Starling MD, MPH, John R. Teerlink MD, Orly Vardeny PharmD, MS, Kazuhiro Yamamoto MD, PhD, Clyde Yancy MD, MSc, Jian Zhang MD, PhD, Shelley Zieroth MD.

Received 2 January 2021, revised 11 January 2021, accepted 13 January 2021, available online 1 March 2021. *Journal of Cardiac Failure* Vol 00 No 00 2021; ScienceDirect (https://www.sciencedirect.com/science/article/pii/S1071916421000506)

Summary of Key Points

In this document, we propose a universal definition of heart failure (HF) as the following: HF is a clinical syndrome with symptoms and or signs caused by a structural and/or functional cardiac abnormality and corroborated by elevated natriuretic peptide levels and/or objective evidence of pulmonary or systemic congestion. We propose revised stages of HF as follows. At-risk for HF (Stage A), for patients at risk for HF but without current or prior symptoms or signs of HF and without structural or biomarkers evidence of heart disease. Pre-HF (stage B), for patients without current or prior symptoms or signs of HF, but evidence of structural heart disease or abnormal cardiac function, or elevated natriuretic peptide levels. HF (Stage C), for patients with current or prior symptoms and/or signs of HF caused by a structural and/or functional cardiac abnormality. Advanced HF (Stage D), for patients with severe symptoms and/or signs of HF at rest, recurrent hospitalizations despite guideline-directed management and therapy (GDMT), refractory or intolerant to GDMT, requiring advanced therapies such as consideration for transplant, mechanical circulatory support or palliative care. Finally, we propose a new and revised classification of HF according to left ventricular ejection fraction (LVEF). The classification includes HF with reduced EF (HFrEF): HF with an LVEF of ≤40%; HF with mildly reduced EF (HFmrEF): HF with an LVEF of 41% to 49%; HF with preserved EF (HFpEF): HF with an LVEF of ≥50%; and HF with improved EF (HFimpEF): HF with a baseline LVEF of ≤40%, a ≥10-point increase from baseline LVEF, and a second measurement of LVEF of >40%.

Gaps in Current Definitions of HF

Combined Definition With Hemodynamic Characterization of HF

The current definitions that include a hemodynamic characterization, such as the HFA/ESC definition, which defines HF as a "a clinical syndrome characterized by typical signs and symptoms, caused by a structural and/or functional cardiac abnormality, resulting in a reduced cardiac output and/or elevated intracardiac pressures at rest or during stress," have the following limitations. Although accurate, this type of definition is hard to apply in public health or epidemiologic settings because of the subjectivity of the symptoms counterbalanced by the unfeasibility (invasive) or unreliability of measurements of cardiac output or filling pressures. For a definition to be also useful for the nonspecialist, it should be assessable easily and with relatively low interobserver variability. The Framingham criteria, which were developed for just such a purpose, are now considered insufficiently specific for adoption as a definition of HF in the contemporary setting.

Proposed New HF Definition

We propose a contemporary universal definition of HF (Figure 1) that is simple but conceptually comprehensive, with near universal applicability, prognostic and therapeutic validity, and acceptable sensitivity and specificity.

universal definition of HF.

HF is a clinical syndrome with current or prior

- Symptoms and or signs caused by a structural and/or functional cardiac abnormality (as determined by an EF of <50%, abnormal cardiac chamber enlargement, E/E' of >15, moderate/severe ventricular hypertrophy or moderate/severe valvular obstructive or regurgitant lesion)

- and corroborated by at least one of the following:

  - Elevated natriuretic peptide levels

  - Objective evidence of cardiogenic pulmonary or systemic congestion by diagnostic modalities, such as imaging (eg, by chest radiograph or elevated filling pressures by echocardiography) or hemodynamic measurement (eg, right heart catheterization, pulmonary artery catheter) at rest or with provocation (eg, exercise)

Proposed Revised Stages of the HF Continuum

To enhance clinician, patient, and public understanding and adoption; to avoid the stigma of HF before the symptoms are manifest; to address the evolving role of biomarkers to define patients with structural and subclinical heart disease who are at higher risk of developing HF and are potential candidates for targeted treatment strategies for the prevention of HF; and to address some of the gaps identified in Section Current Classification According to Stages of HF and Its Limitations in the current approach to staging HF, we propose the following stages.

- **AT RISK FOR HF (STAGE A):** Patients at risk for HF, but without current or prior symptoms or signs of HF and without structural cardiac changes or elevated biomarkers of heart disease. Patients with hypertension, atherosclerotic cardiovascular disease, diabetes, obesity, known exposure to cardiotoxins, a positive family history of cardiomyopathy, or genetic cardiomyopathy would be in this category. Not all of these patients will develop HF, but risk factor intervention may be warranted.

- **PRE-HF (STAGE B):** Patients without current or prior symptoms or signs of HF with evidence of one of the following:

- Structural Heart Disease: for example, left ventricular hypertrophy, cardiac chamber enlargement, ventricular wall motion abnormality, myocardial tissue abnormality (eg, evidence of myocardial edema, scar/fibrosis abnormality by T2-weighted cardiac magnetic resonance imaging or late gadolinium enhancement imaging), valvular heart disease.

- Abnormal cardiac function: for example, reduced left or right ventricular systolic function, evidence of increased filling pressures (by invasive or noninvasive measures), abnormal diastolic dysfunction.

- Elevated natriuretic peptide levels or elevated cardiac troponin levels (>99th percentile in a normal reference population), especially in the setting of exposure to cardiotoxins.

- **HF (STAGE C):** Patients with current or prior symptoms and/or signs of hf caused by a structural and/or functional cardiac abnormality.

- **ADVANCED HF (STAGE D):** Severe symptoms and/or signs of HF at rest, recurrent hospitalizations despite GDMT, refractory or intolerant to GDMT, requiring advanced therapies such as consideration for transplantation, mechanical circulatory support, or palliative care.

Proposed New Classifications of HF According to EF

The strongest argument to use LVEF to categorize HF is that LVEF defines a group known to respond to life-prolonging therapy from randomized controlled trials. Although the LVEF also provides prognostic information, this reason alone does not justify using LVEF to define HF. Accordingly, LVEF categories were created that define groups where treatment differs.

To be able to differentiate patients who benefit from GDMT according to clinical trial entry criteria of patients with HFrEF, capture evolving recognition of the need to identify effective treatment strategies in patients with HF associated with a mildly reduced or mid-range LVEF, as well as preserved LVEF, and harmonize with existing practice guidelines, we propose the following four classifications of EF

- **HF with reduced EF (HFrEF):** HF with LVEF ≤40%.

- **HF with mildly reduced EF (HFmrEF):** HF with LVEF 41-49%

- **HF with preserved EF (HFpEF):** HF with LVEF ≥50%.

- **HF with improved EF (HFimpEF):** HF with a baseline LVEF of ≤40%, a ≥10-point increase from baseline LVEF, and a second measurement of LVEF of >40%.

Perspective for the Non-cardiologist

The majority of the HF care is provided by noncardiologists, including general practitioners, internal medicine or family medicine clinicians, hospitalists, emergency room providers, and other specialists. We believe the universal definition will be useful to these clinicians for the timely diagnosis and management of patients with HF. Important points for the noncardiologists are as follows. It is critical to optimally identify and treat patients at risk for HF to prevent or delay the development of HF; recognize that pre-HF patients, such as asymptomatic patients with elevated natriuretic peptide levels likely will require referral to a cardiologist for further diagnostic and treatment strategies to prevent progression of HF; that the diagnosis and timely treatment of HF should not be missed or delayed in patients with symptoms and signs of HF; and that elevated natriuretic peptide levels or patients with evidence of systemic or pulmonary congestion/elevated filling pressures, and patients with advanced HF would be considered for referral to HF specialists according to their goals.

NEW DEFINITION

HF is a clinical syndrome with current or prior

- **Symptoms and or signs caused by a structural and/or functional cardiac abnormality** (as determined by an EF of <50%, abnormal cardiac chamber enlargement, E/E' of >15, moderate/severe ventricular hypertrophy or moderate/severe valvular obstructive or regurgitant lesion)

- and **corroborated by** at least one of the following:
  - *Elevated natriuretic peptide levels*
  - *Objective evidence* of cardiogenic pulmonary or systemic congestion by diagnostic modalities, such as imaging (eg, by chest radiograph or elevated filling pressures by echocardiography) or hemodynamic measurement (eg, right heart catheterization, pulmonary artery catheter) at rest or with provocation (eg, exercise)

the Consensus Statement was published by *Journal of Cardiac Failure* Vol 27 No 4 2021 (see reference, page 11)

List of illustrations, tables and photographs

the heart as two pumps 23
the pathway of blood flow through the heart 24
the coronary tree as seen on cardiac CT imaging.............. 25
blood vessels wrapped around the heart............................. 26
the electrical system 27
the valves within the heart 28
gas exchange 29
fluid within the body... 30
a sick heart... 32
consequences of cardiac failure.. 33
understanding ejection fraction: how EF is determined 36
ejection fraction... 39
understanding cardiac output 40
the circulatory system...41
the respiratory system 41
journey of the blood... 42
layers of the heart 44
circle of circulation 45
the kidneys...49
filtration system: swimming pool analogy 50
filtration system: body's renal system..............................51
nephron anatomy 52
the lungs in relation to the heart 53
Terry...55
maintaining fluid balance and blood pressure................... 58
receptors 58
the cerebral cortex 59
tensions within the heart... 62
the kidneys are the filtration system of the body 63
renin-angiotensin-aldosterone system (RAAS).................. 64
the heart can change structurally...................................... 68
the sympathetic nervous system/the para sympathetic
    nervous system.. 69
Emma and Peter 73
when a valve doesn't work 93
New York Heart Association (NYHA) Classification of
    Cardiac Failure 102
heart sounds 104
ECG trace that shows a heart under strain 106

an x-ray showing Kerley B lines 107
echocardiogram, showing the heart structure and valves in
    a healthy heart in diastole and systole 110
    a dilated heart in diastole and systole 111
is the problem regional or global? 112
cardiac imaging: invasive angiogram, CT angiogram,
    cardiac magnetic resonance...115
Kathleen's well-kept graph 121
Kathleen...123
kidney detail 133
kidney refresher: pool analogy 134
kidney refresher: the body 135
understanding diuretics 138
understanding ACE inhibitors 143
bilateral renal artery stenosis (RAS) 149
disaster..152
autonomic nervous system...156
a pacemaker..170
an implantable cardiac defibrillator...170
chambers of the heart..172
a deliberate hole in the heart? 178
implantation of a stent 179
mitral stenosis/ mitral incompetence 180
aortic stenosis/aortic incompetence 181
Gordon, after heart surgery...184
Gordon, enjoying his new life..187
takotsubo 211
Cam and family..219
exercise letter from a patient..223
drugs of cardiac failure...254
timelines 256
action of agent 258
electrical activity in a normal heart..260
the heart and an ECG...262
sinus rhythm as shown on an ECG 263
universal definition of HF...268

Glossary

A

abnormalities

global – a problem that affects all of the heart

regional – a problem that affects only part of the heart; for example, scar tissue after a heart attack

afferent arteriole

takes blood to the glomerulus (in the kidney)

aldosterone

a mineralocorticoid produced in the renin-angiotensin-aldosterone system (RAAS) that acts at the distal tubule, retaining sodium and therefore water, thus keeping up the fluid level

aldosterone blocker/antagonist

blocks the renin-angiotensin-aldosterone system (RAAS), releasing sodium and water, which then passes from the body as urine; most commonly used drugs are spironolactone and eplerenone

amyloidosis

amyloid protein infiltrates the heart muscle, thickens it, making it stiff and unable to pump correctly

angiogram

contrast (die) injected into a patient that outlines the coronary arteries in explicit detail, giving information about the location, the quality and nature of the plaque, the degree of stenosis and the size of the vessel affected. There are two types of coronary angiogram. One is often referred to as CT coronary angiogram or a CCTA, a coronary computed tomography angiogram, which is non-invasive. The other is 'invasive' and requires a small tube to be passed from an artery in the arm or leg into the heart so that dye can be injected directly into the coronary arteries.

angiotensin II (AT2)

works on the angiotensin II receptor and causes vasoconstriction – keeps up the blood pressure; constricts the kidney's efferent arteriole and so increases filtration. The resultant fluid overload places a strain on the heart that could be detrimental to a heart in cardiac failure.

angiotensin II (AT2) receptor

drives much of the action within the renin-angiotensin-aldosterone system (RAAS), including the production of aldosterone

angiotensin II (AT2) receptor blocker (ARB)

acts directly on the AT2 receptor in the renin-angiotensin-aldosterone system (RAAS), releasing sodium and water, which then passes from the body as urine; lowers blood pressure, relaxes efferent arteriole, lessens aldosterone production. Commonly used drugs are candesartan and valsartan. Should not be given with ACE inhibitors, although they are interchangeable.

angiotensin-converting enzyme (ACE)

the enzyme that converts angiotensin I (AT1) to angiotensin II (AT2)

angiotensin-converting enzyme (ACE) inhibitor

blocks the renin-angiotensin-aldosterone system (RAAS) – prevents the conversion of AT1 to AT2 – releasing sodium and water, which then passes from the body as urine. Used for patients whose hearts are not pumping well – hearts with reduced ejection fraction (HFrEF). Current commonly used drugs include enalapril, perindopril and ramipril. Should not be given with ARBs, although they are interchangeable.

angiotensin-converting enzyme (ACE) inhibitor side-effects

blood pressure, kidney function, aldosterone levels, cough; need ongoing monitoring

atrial fibrillation (AF)
an 'irregularly irregular' heartbeat, characterized by the loss of the coordinated contraction of the top part of the heart, the atrial chambers, or atria. It affects the pumping capacity of the heart. The condition can be managed but not cured.

atrial flutter
a rapid and regular rhythm arising from the right side of the heart

arteries
the vessels of the body's circulatory system that carry blood away from the heart

ascites
fluid in the abdomen

associations
connected, joined or related to

asymptomatic
producing or showing no symptoms

atrium
a pre-pumping chamber of the heart. There is an atrium on each side of the heart – the right atrium helps move blood from the body into the right ventricle and to the lungs; the left atrium helps move blood from the lungs into the left ventricle (the main pumping chamber of the heart) and into the body

autonomic nervous system (ANS)
the nerve function that occurs without us giving the action a thought; it is automatic

   sympathetic nervous system (SNS) prepares the body for 'fight or flight' response; kicks in when the body is challenged; like an accelerator in a car

   parasympathetic nervous system (PNS) helps the body slow down, to 'digest and relax'; like a brake in a car

B

barometric pressure
the pressure within the fluid of the vasculature of the body's large blood vessels

baroreceptors
pressure receptors that measure the barometric pressure. They are found in two locations within the body, the aortic arch and the carotid arteries.

beta-blockers / beta blockade
dampen the over-drive effect of the sympathetic nervous system; target the high density of beta receptors (specifically beta2 receptors) in the heart; commonly used drugs are carvedilol, bisoprolol, extended-release metoprolol and nebivolol; improves mortality, morbidity and quality of life for people with reduced cardiac function

beta-blocker side-effects
lowered blood pressure, fatigue, can worsen asthma

beta receptors
part of the receptor system that regulates the body's response to the sympathetic nervous system

bicuspid aortic valve
has two leaflets instead of the standard three; present from birth (*see also* valve, aortic)

bilateral renal artery stenosis (RAS)
narrowing of both renal arteries causing a significant impairment to blood flow to the two kidneys, simultaneously; a rare condition

biopsy
small piece tissue is put under a microscope to investigate at a cellular level; a possible, but not standard, test

bisoprolol
a commonly-use beta-blocker; others include carvedilol, extended-release metoprolol and nebivolol

bi-ventricular pacemaker
see resynchronization

blood
the fluid that transports cells, oxygen and nutrients to the body and removes carbon dioxide and other waste

blood clot (thrombosis)
formation of a blood clot is a normal response to prevent bleeding when damage occurs to a blood vessel wall. A soft, thick clump of platelets and fibrin forms to 'plug' a hole in an artery or vein to prevent blood loss. Very dangerous. They can lead to major disasters such as stroke, pulmonary embolism, deep vein thrombosis (DVT), kidney failure and pregnancy complications.

blood flow restoration
procedures to restore blood flow to blocked arteries include the implantation of a stent/s or bypass grafting

BNP (B-type natriuretic peptide or brain natriuretic peptide)
a discriminating test to help clarify if there is a problem with the heart or if the shortness of breath is related to something other than the heart

bypass graft
used to restore blood flow to the heart; a piece of 'tube', from an artery or vein, is used to take blood around the blockage/s to healthier arteries so that good blood flow reaches the heart muscle

C

calcium channel blockers
blood pressure agents best avoided in the presence of cardiac failure

candesartan
a commonly used AT2 receptor blocker (ARB); can be used for blood pressure. Valsartan is another commonly used ARB.

captopril
the first of the angiotensin-converting enzyme (ACE-I) inhibitors, a powerful agent developed in the 1990s for the treatment and management of congestive heart failure in people with decreased LV function, or reduced contraction of the heart. Its use provided improved quality of life, morbidity and mortality.

cardiac contractility modulation
a new procedure that alters the way calcium in the cells of the heart is utilized, increasing the effectiveness of the muscle contraction; also alters phosphorylation; has been approved for use in the United States by the US Food and Drug Administration and is currently under review in other jurisdictions, including Australia

cardiac failure (CF)
the heart does not pump as well as it should, leading to a complex mix of a sick heart, maladapted responses to impaired circulation and fluid retention that further strains the heart into a downward spiral of deterioration

cardiac failure, acute
when the heart fails suddenly; a medical emergency

cardiac failure, classifications
time – acute or chronic

function – ejection fraction, reduced or preserved

degree of incapacity brought on by breathlessness – the New York Heart Association Classification of Cardiac Failure (NYHA)

cardiac failure, types
left ventricular (LV), the left-hand side of the heart has impaired function

HF with Reduced Ejection Fraction (HFrEF) – LV does not contract properly

HF with Preserved Ejection Fraction (HFpEF) – LV loses its ability to relax

right-sided heart failure (often a result of left-side failure) fluid pressure, backed up through the lungs, causes the right side of the heart to compensate, then eventually decompensate

cardiac imaging
any method used to image the muscle, valves and arteries of the heart
echocardiography – assesses dynamic function of muscle and valves

CT imaging – assesses the health of the arteries in a non-invasive way

invasive angiography – provides a clear picture of the narrowing of the arteries

magnetic resonance imaging (MRI)/ cardiac magnetic resonance (CMR) – shows scarring within the heart and inflammation, in exquisite detail

nuclear medicine – assesses aspects of cellular function

cardiac output
the volume of blood pumped per minute

cardiomyopathy
a disease of the heart muscle

dilated – when there is systolic failure and the ejection fraction is   lessened

infiltrative – by-products of the body's metabolism accumulate within the body's tissues and infiltrate the heart tissues causing a loss of function

hypertrophic – abnormal genes cause the heart muscle to grow thick

tachycardia-induced – the cardiomyopathy is caused by a long-term fast heart rate

cardiovascular disease (CVD)
general term for conditions affecting the heart or blood vessels; includes coronary heart disease, angina, heart attack, congenital heart disease, stroke and vascular dementia

carvedilol
a commonly-used beta-blocker; others include bisoprolol, extended-release metoprolol and nebivolol

causations
factors/actions that cause the problem

circulatory system
works with the respiratory system to move blood and so, oxygen/carbon dioxide throughout the body; this system connects the heart, the kidneys and the lungs to all organs

co-morbidities
other serious conditions suffered concurrently with the primary health problem

crepitations
fine, crackly sounds in the lungs (like gently scrunched cellophane) heard when the patient is suffering heart failure

D

dapagliflozin
sodium-glucose transport inhibitor (SGLT2 inhibitor); *see* gliflozin

depression
an association of cardiac failure; found in about 20 percent of CF suffers; worsens CF prognosis and worsens quality of life

diastole
relaxation phase of heart function (*see also* ejection fraction)

digoxin
derived from the foxglove plant, and used for hundreds of years, a drug for slowing the heart rate by acting on the AV node, thus slowing the ventricle; improves the contractility of the heart muscle

dilated cardiomyopathy
dilated, the ventricle is bigger than it should be; *cardio*, the heart; *myo* muscle; *pathy*, disease *see* cardiomyopathy

dilated left atrium
enlarged pre-pump chamber on the left side of the heart

diltiazem
a calcium channel blocker that should be avoided in the presence of cardiac failure; *also* verapamil

disease
a symptom or loss of normal function

distal
situated away from the center

diuretic
medication to make a patient pass fluid – relieves congestion and reduces strain on the heart

diuretic, loop
medication that works by blocking the concentrating mechanisms within the loop of the renal tubule, the Loop of Henle; the most used drug is furosemide

E

echocardiogram (echo)
echo, sound, *cardio*, heart, *gram*, picture
a scan of the heart using ultra sound waves to acquire a picture. It gives information about the valves, the chambers of the heart and pressures within the heart

efferent arteriole
takes blood away from the glomerulus (in the kidney)

ejection fraction (EF)
refers to the amount of blood ejected or expelled from the left ventricle (LV), the main pumping chamber of the heart, with each heartbeat, expressed as a percentage of the total volume of blood contained within the LV. It indicates how well the LV is working.

> reduced EF (HFrEF), systolic failure (the heart does not contract properly and so it does not push out as much blood as it should), less than 50 percent

> preserved EF (HFpEF) diastolic failure (the heart contracts normally but fails to relax, limiting the LV' s refilling ability; resulting in a stiff or thickened heart muscle), 50 percent or higher

electrocardiogram (ECG)
a trace of the electrical activity through the heart acquired by electrodes. It shows the rhythm of the heart. Features of an ECG can be used to determine the status of the heart muscle.

empagliflozin
a gliflozin or sodium-glucose transport inhibitor (SGLT2 inhibitor)

enalapril
one of the ACE inhibitor drugs currently used in the treatment and management of congestive heart failure in people with decreased LV function, or reduced contraction of the heart; providing improved quality of life, morbidity and mortality; other similar drugs include perindopril and ramipril

eplerenone
a common aldosterone antagonist that works on the distal tubule

erythropoietin (EPO)
hormone produced by the kidneys to stimulate the production of red blood cells; should not be used as a treatment for anemia in association with cardiac failure as stimulating red blood cell growth can lead to increased clotting

extra corporeal membrane oxygenation (ECMO)
a machine, very similar to a bypass machine, takes blood from the patient to transfer oxygen through a membrane outside the body to maintain oxygenation to the person; used for critically unwell patients with a good chance of recovery

F

fluid balance
the sweet spot between fluid over-load and under-load

> 'too wet', which presents as shortness of breath, swollen ankles and weight gain

> 'too dry', which presents as light-headedness from too little fluid in the circulation, thirst, dry skin, and dark urine from an increased concentration of fluid

fluid tablets
see diuretics

furosemide
one of the most commonly used loop diuretic drugs

G

gliflozin
sodium-glucose transport inhibitor (SGLT2 inhibitor) that works at the proximal tubule of the kidney, allowing salt and water to be lost through the urine; developed initially to aid diabetics; reduces hospitalizations, improves quality of life especially for diabetic patients with CF, improves mortality drug; the most used drug is empagliflozin, while a 2019 report to the European Society of Cardiology showed that the drug, dapagliflozin, was a beneficial add-on therapy for cardiac failure patients already appropriately treated regardless of whether or not they had diabetes

glomerulus
a cluster of tiny blood cells forming the filter within each kidney

H

heart
the muscle organ that pumps blood through the body

heart attack
a non-medical expression (a layman's term) referring to a major heart problem; most commonly, but not always, caused by the narrowing of the coronary arteries that can kill or requires some form of medical intervention – medication, time in hospital, stents, or coronary artery bypass grafting to restore the blood flow to the muscle

heart transplant
the patient is given a new heart from a donor; first performed in the world at Groote Schuur Hospital, Cape Town, South Africa, by Dr Christiaan Barnard on 3 December 1967

HFpEF, HFrEF
see ejection fraction

homeostasis
homeo, similar; *stasis*, being stable; *homeostasis*, the capacity of the body to maintain stability of diverse internal variables the maintenance of the body's pre-set determinants such as blood pressure, heart rate, digestion, and kidney filtration

hibernating myocardium
the middle layer of heart tissue (myocardium) becomes dormant from lack of adequate blood supply but functions normally again once the blood flow has been restored

hydralazine
a direct smooth muscle relaxant that reduces blood pressure; an older drug now used for people who do not tolerate ACE inhibitors or the AT2 receptor blockers

I

implantable cardiac defibrillator (ICD)
a battery powered device sitting under the clavicle with 'wires' placed in the heart to monitor rhythm and detect irregular heartbeats; delivers a shock to the heart to re-establish normal rhythm if the heart develops a potentially fatal rhythm (goes into cardiac arrest); can be used in conjunction with resynchronization therapy; highly specialized

intra-aortic balloon pump (IABP)
highly specialised, mechanical option for treatment in an acute setting; a balloon, placed in the aorta, expands and contracts, synchronized with the heartbeat, making it easier for the heart to pump; needs to be timed meticulously to the individual's heartbeat

ivabradine
works at the sinus node of the right atrium to slow down the heart rate; improves symptomatic control

K

Kerley B lines
fine lines within the lungs, as seen on x-ray, that correspond to the crepitations heard when a patient is suffering CF

kidneys
bean-shaped primary organs of the body's renal system; the body's 'treatment plant'; have essential role in CF as they maintain fluid balance throughout the circulatory system and also maintain salt and mineral levels within the body, which affect blood pressure

L

layers of the heart

pericardium – *peri*, around; *cardium*, heart outside covering

endocardium – endo, inner; *cardium*, heart inner surface of the heart's chambers

left atrium decompression

a new procedure still under investigation; for people who have heart failure with preserved ejection fraction (HFpEF), in which the pressure in the left atrium generally increases, transmitting the pressure backwards into the lungs and forward into the left ventricle. Research shows that a hole could be made between the left atrium and the right atrium so that the blood drains from the left side to the right side, thus decompressing the left atrium.

left bundle branch block (LBBB)

electrical impulses that activate the heart muscle pass through the heart in a discordant manner – through the muscle cells rather than through the Purkinje fibres; reduces heart's co-ordination which reduces its efficiency

left ventricular assist device (LVAD)

an external device that works in conjunction with the patient's own heart; used in the end stages of heart failure to keep the person alive until possible transplant

Loop of Henle

a region between the proximal and distal tubules of the kidney where concentration of urine may occur; a region where certain diuretic drugs (loop diuretics) work

lungs

two sponge-like, interdependent organs connected by the circulation. They are located on either side of the chest (thorax) and close to the heart. The life-giving carbon dioxide/oxygen exchange takes place in the lungs.

J

juxtaglomerular apparatus

juxta, near*; glomerulus*, filtration unit; *apparatus*, a collection of specialised cells

regulates body fluid from within the kidneys responding to local BP and input from the autonomic nervous system. It acts on the renin-angiotensin-aldosterone system (RAAS) so that the body retains fluid, keeps sodium and water in the kidneys and stimulates the sympathetic nervous system to increase blood pressure by constructing the arteries.

M

metoprolol

a commonly used beta-blocker; others include bisoprolol, carvedilol and nebivolol; available in an extended-release preparation for CF

mineralocorticoid

corticoids, steroid-based hormones; *mineralo*, mineral balance)

hormone messengers that influence electrolyte and water balance in the body; the primary mineralocorticoid is aldosterone

mineralocorticoid blocker

can be used as a diuretic. If used in conjunction with a loop diuretic, particular care needs to be exercised around fluid balance and fluid loss, with regular blood testing and clinical assessment essential.

moxonidine

a blood pressure agent that is not beneficial for cardiac failure patients

myocardium

myo, muscle, *cardio*, being of the heart the muscle of the heart

N

natriuretic peptide system (NPS)

the chemical messenger system that protects the heart

nebivolol

a commonly used beta-blocker; others include bisoprolol, carvedilol and extended-release metoprolol

neprilysin inhibitor

helps stop the breakdown of the natriuretic peptides (good guys); cannot be used in conjunction with ACE inhibitors; commonly use drug, sacubitril

New York Heart Association Classification of Cardiac Failure (NYHA)

a set of guidelines based on the impact impaired breathing has on a patient; brings commonality to discussions across medical disciplines

nephron

the blood filtering unit within the kidneys (which includes the filter, the glomerulus). There are about one million nephrons in each kidney.

neural

nerve-based response

neurohumoral

neuro, nerves; *humoral*, messengers within the blood

nitrates

a direct smooth muscle relaxant that works on the venous system to reduce the blood flow back to the heart, so 'offloading' the heart; an older drug now used for people who do not tolerate ACE inhibitors or the AT2 receptor blockers

non-steroidal anti-inflammatory drug (NSAID)

reduces the production of chemical messengers, prostaglandins, responsible for inflammatory responses within the body. Great for aches and pains but can precipitate renal failure (a disaster) if used in association with an ACE inhibitor or an AT2 blocker – the NSAID constricts the afferent arteriole while the ACE inhibitor or the AT2 blocker relaxes the efferent arteriole. Commonly used NSAIDs are Nurofen and Voltaren.

P

perindopril

one of the ACE inhibitor drugs currently used in the treatment and management of congestive heart failure in people with decreased LV function, or reduced contraction of the heart; providing improved quality of life, morbidity and mortality; other similar drugs include enalapril and ramipril

peripheral edema

peripheral, arms and legs; *edema*, swelling fluid in the legs

potassium

a salt in balance with sodium; can act as a vasodilator to lower the risk of high blood pressure

preserved EF (HFpEF)

see ejection fraction

prognostic (prognosis)

the long-term outcome for the patient

proximal

situated near the center

pulmonary artery blood pressure monitoring

requires a small device to be implanted into the pulmonary trunk; gives a good indication of how pressures and blood flow could be loading the lungs and the heart; used for critical and acute patients in intensive care units; has not been taken up widely for outpatients

pulse

a beat felt under the skin from the contraction of the left ventricle, which makes the blood flow through the body's arteries. It can be felt in several locations including the wrist and the neck. In a healthy heart, the pulse is strong and regular.

R

ramipril

one of the ACE inhibitor drugs currently used in the treatment and management of congestive heart failure in people with decreased LV function, or reduced contraction of the heart; providing improved quality of life, morbidity and mortality; other similar drugs include enalapril and perindopril

receptors

the means by which hormones or chemical messengers in the bloodstream interact with their target cells. A receptor is simply a 'docking station' that is specific to the hormone or chemical in question.

renal artery

transports blood into each kidney

renal vein

returns blood to the body

renin-angiotensin-aldosterone system (RAAS)

the chemical messenger system that regulates blood pressure through the kidneys; produces aldosterone (keeps sodium in the kidneys – increases fluid volume in the body)

renin-angiotensin-aldosterone system (RAAS) blocker

releases sodium and water, which pass out of the body as urine. Therapies include angiotensin-converting enzyme (ACE) inhibitors, angiotensin II (AT2) receptor blockers, aldosterone blockers

reduced EF (HFrEF)

see ejection fraction

respiratory system

works with the circulatory system to move blood and oxygen/carbon dioxide throughout the body

resynchronization therapy

re-establishes synchronicity within the heart by using a special pacemaker – a bi-ventricular pacemaker – that can overcome the time delay of a bundle branch block; can be used in association with an implantable cardiac defibrillator; highly specialized; improves symptoms, heart function and quality of life

rhythm

> sinus (normal) – the healthy heart rhythm, which is controlled by the sinoatrial or sinus node beating in a synchronistic and smooth manner

> arrhythmia – when the synchronicity of the heartbeat breaks down

S

sacubitril

clinically-available neprilysin inhibitor, available as a combination medication with an AT2 receptor blocker

salt/sodium

associated with fluid retention and elevation of blood pressure

shortness of breath

a symptom of CF

> orthopnea – *ortho*, upright; *pnea,* breathing

> shortness of breath while in a recumbent position

> paroxysmal nocturnal dyspnea (PND), shortness of breath that comes unexpectedly in the middle of the night, accompanied by a feeling of suffocation which provokes anxiety and fear; a precursor to orthopnea

sodium-glucose transport inhibitor (SGLT2)

see gliflozin

spironolactone

a common aldosterone antagonist that works on the distal tubule in each kidney

stenosis

narrowing

stenting

mechanical intervention for coronary artery disease in which an intravascular device (balloon) within a wire scaffold is inserted percutaneously (through the skin) and guided to the site of the narrowing. When the balloon is inflated, the artery is opened. When the balloon is removed, the wire scaffold remains to keep the artery open. The scaffold is called a stent.

stroke
a disruption of the blood supply to the brain, leading to permanent loss of function

> hemorrhagic – when a blood vessel ruptures and bleeds into the brain

> ischemic – when a clot blocks an artery, leading to a lack of blood flow

systole
see ejection fraction

T

takotsubo
broken heart syndrome; brought on by emotional stress; the sympathetic nervous system discharges so much nervous energy that it shuts down the heart; the symptoms are similar to a heart attack, but the person does not have blocked arteries

transcutaneous aortic valve implantation (TAVI)
minimally invasive technology to replace a stenosed aortic valve

troponin
protein found in the heart that is leaked into the blood when the heart is damaged or stressed. A blood test to measure the troponin level is used as a predictor when a person presents with chest pain to assess the likelihood of the heart being involved

U

ultrafiltration
highly specialised, mechanical option for treatment; sucks fluid out of the circulatory system using a process similar to dialysis; Does not require drugs; does not need the kidneys to be functioning well

V

valsartan
a commonly used AT2 receptor blocker (ARB); can be used for blood pressure. Candesartan is another commonly used ARB.

valves (in order of blood flow)
the heart has four valves that keep blood flowing in the correct direction; each valve has flaps (leaflets or cusps) that open and close once during each heartbeat

> tricuspid – a one-way valve between the right atrium and the right ventricle

> pulmonary – a one-way valve between the right ventricle and the pulmonary circulation that takes the carbon dioxide-saturated blood from the heart to the lungs

> mitral – a one-way valve between the left atrium and the left ventricle

> aortic – a one-way valve between the left ventricle and the aorta, which is the main artery of the body and takes oxygen-rich blood from the heart to the organs and tissues of the body

valve repair/replacement
the mitral valve and the aortic valve, both on the left side of the heart, can become too tight (stenosis) or leak (regurgitation or incompetence).

> mitral valve can be repaired (preferred) or replaced using metallic or biological tissue

> aortic valve can be replaced either by open heart surgery or for a tight aortic valve, by minimally-invasive technology called transcutaneous aortic valve implantation (TAVI)

vasoconstriction
a tightening of the blood vessel which increases tension within the vessel and keeps up the blood pressure

veins

blood vessels that mostly carry deoxygenated blood towards the heart. The ones that most concern us are:

IVC – inferior vena cava is one of two major veins that drains into the right atrium; it collects blood flowing below the heart

jugular – carries blood from the brain, face and neck, and connects with the SVC to take the blood to the right atrium; a 'dipstick' for fluid pressure in the right atrium (the waveform of the jugular pulse is often visible in patients with a sick heart when sitting upright)

pulmonary – is one of the exceptions, and the four pulmonary veins transfer oxygenated blood from the lungs to the left atrium of the heart

SVC – superior vena cava is one of two major veins that drains into the right atrium; it collects blood flowing above the heart.

ventricle

the main compression (pumping) chamber of the heart that pushes the blood through the body. There is a right and the left ventricle. The right ventricle pumps the oxygen-poor blood into the lungs while the left ventricle (the main pumping chamber of the heart) pumps oxygen-rich blood into the body.

verapamil

a calcium channel blocker that should be avoided in the presence of cardiac failure; *also* diltiazem

viable heart muscle

heart muscle that is not receiving enough blood but is still alive
(see also hibernating myocardium)

X

xenotransplantation

process of grafting or transplanting organs, tissues or cells between different animal species

Index

A

abnormalities
  global, 110, 112, 273, 274

  regional, 110, 111, 112, 162, 163, 273, 274

aldosterone (includes blocker/antagonist) 35, 57, 58, 62, 64-70, 132, 136-138, 140, 141, 142, 143, 145, 147, 148, 154, 159, 160, 165, 192, 250, 254, 256, 272, 274, 278, 280, 282

amyloidosis 88, 90-92, 274

angiogram 115, 163, 174, 209, 212, 273, 274

angiotensin (includes I and II, At1, AT2, blocker, receptor, receptor blocker) 62, 64-70, 80, 130, 132, 141, 143, 144, 145, 146, 147-150, 151, 152, 154, 160, 161, 165, 167, 168, 192, 218, 234, 250,254, 272, 274, 276, 279, 280, 281, 282, 283

angiotensin-converting enzyme (includes ACE, ACE inhibitor, ACE inhibitor side-effects) 6, 64, 65, 66, 70, 80, 92, 119, 132, 140, 141-145, 147, 148, 149, 150, 151, 152, 154, 160, 161, 164, 165, 167, 168, 174, 175, 193, 194, 218, 235, 236, 243, 250, 254, 256, 257, 258, 273, 274, 276, 278, 279, 281, 282

angiotensinogen 64, 65, 70

arteriole/s 45, 47
  afferent 51, 63, 134, 135, 151, 258, 274, 281

  efferent 51, 63, 64, 66, 135, 141, 142, 147, 148, 151, 258, 274, 278, 281

artery and arteries are used extensively throughout the book. More specific references include
  coronary artery disease 15, 21, 32, 34, 85, 96, 114, 127, 179, 189, 196, 211, 225, 232, 242, 282, 286

  carotid 16, 43, 61, 69, 184, 275

  pulmonary 23, 24, 28, 43, 48, 131, 176, 189, 268, 271, 281

  renal 51, 52, 134, 149, 273, 275, 282

atrial fibrillation (AF) 28, 32, 34, 56, 95, 96, 103, 166, 168, 191, 192, 193, 203, 204 (fn), 209, 224, 229 (fn), 275, 287

ascites 105, 275

asymptomatic 56, 271, 275

atrium/atria (includes left, right) 22, 23, 24, 26, 27, 28, 30, 39, 41, 43, 46, 47, 48, 86, 97, 98, 104, 109, 130, 130, 131, 138, 161, 165, 168, 172, 178, 189, 192, 194, 221, 260, 261, 262, 275, 277, 279, 280, 283, 284

autonomic nervous system (ANS) 32, 35, 57, 59-62, 69, 155, 156, 159, 192, 211, 243, 245, 273, 275, 280

B

barometric pressure 61, 275

baroreceptors 61, 65, 69, 275

beta-blocker/s (includes blockade, receptors, side-effects) 92, 130, 132, 154,55-158, 164, 175, 176, 192, 194, 211, 218, 235, 236, 242, 250, 254, 255, 275, 277, 280, 281

bicuspid aortic valve 162, 163, 165, 275

bilateral renal artery stenosis (RAS) 6, 149, 273, 275

biopsy 109, 116, 275

bisoprolol 75, 92, 156, 175, 236, 254, 257, 275, 277, 280, 281

bi-ventricular pacemaker 171, 176, 189, 257, 275

blood flow restoration 131, 276

BNP (B-type natriuretic peptide, brain natriuretic peptide / natriuretic peptide/s) 98, 109, 113-114, 116, 159, 160, 167, 196, 206, 234, 276, 281

bypass graft/s/ing 179, 189, 276, 279

C

calcium channel blocker 192, 276, 277, 284

candesartan 147, 254, 274, 276, 283

captopril 141, 254, 276

cardiac contractility modulation 131, 177, 189, 276

cardiac failure / heart failure used extensively throughout the book. More specific references include
cardiac failure at a glance 77-78

cardiac failure
acute 78, 101, 205-213, 127, 199, 205, 256, 276, 279, 281

chronic 78, 101, 127, 128, 132, 199, 229 (fn), 256, 276

cardiac failure
classifications
timing
acute, 10, 78, 101, 127, 199, 202, 205-213, 256, 276, 279

chronic, 10, 78, 101, 127, 199

function
ejection fraction, reduced *see ejection fraction*

ejection fraction, preserved *see ejection fraction*

the New York Heart Association Classification of Cardiac Failure (NYHA) 78, 83, 101, 102, 119, 122, 272, 276, 281

types
left ventricular (LV)
HF with Reduced Ejection Fraction (HFrEF) 77

HF with Preserved Ejection Fraction (HFpEF) 77

right-sided heart failure 77, 270

cardiac/coronary imaging, 109, 114-115, 163, 273, 276
echocardiography/echocardiogram 38, 56, 75, 76, 98, 109–110, 113-114, 116, 163, 164, 174, 193, 194, 209, 235, 237, 244, 256, 257, 268, 271, 273, 276, 278

CT imaging 114, 115, 273

invasive angiography 115, 273

magnetic resonance imaging (MRI)/ cardiac magnetic resonance (CMR) 114, 115, 273,277

nuclear medicine 38, 91, 277

cardiac output
31, 32, 40, 85, 86, 94, 96, 155, 267, 277

cardiomyopathy
dilated, 40, 88, 162, 163, 164, 165, 219, 244, 248, 257, 277

genetic, 269

hypertrophic, 89, 277

infiltrative, 89, 277

non-ischemic, 171

tachycardia-induced, 193, 194, 195, 277

takotsubo, 210-11

cardiovascular disease (CVD) 8, 21, 78, 269, 277

carvedilol 156, 164, 254, 275, 277, 280, 281

circulation 15, 16-17, 29, 30, 35, 38, 41, (41-46), 45, 47, 51, 77, 80, 82, 88, 93, 94, 98, 128, 135, 139, 141, 159, 176, 189, 206, 207, 208, 209, 272, 276, 278, 280, 283

circulatory system 25, 30, 41, (41-46), 43, 49, 53, 54, 66, 85, 94, 98, 160, 208, 272, 277, 279, 282, 283

co-morbidities 38, 39, 126, 217, 277

crepitations 105, 107, 277, 279

D

dapagliflozin 167, 168 (fn), 277, 279

depression 16, 32, 33, 199, 200, 201, 203, 224, 233, 257, 277

diabetes/diabetic/s 8, 38, 39, 98, 99, 166, 167, 168, 191, 197, 217, 232, 269, 279, 286

diastole/diastolic 36, 37, 38, 47, 71, 86, 88, 91, 93, 96, 105, 109, 110, 111, 112, 232, 269, 273, 277, 278

digoxin 130, 132, 159, 166, 168, 194, 249, 250, 254, 277

dilated left atrium 97, 277

diltiazem 192, 277, 284

diuretic/s, fluid tablets /loop 13, 14, 79, 80, 83, 92, 99, 119, 120, 121, 128, 129, 130, 132, (133-140), 133, 138, 139, 140, 152, 153, 164, 166, 175, 197, 207, 213, 233, 236, 240, 245, 249, 250, 254, 256, 258, 273, 277, 278, 280

E

echocardiogram (echo)
see cardiac imaging

ejection fraction (EF) 35–39, 40, 47, 78, 91, 92, 98, 99, 109,12, 127, 128, 131, 163, 169, 171, 173, 174, 175, 192, 194, 195, 234, 235, 237, 267, 272, 276, 277, 278, 279, 283

preserved, EF (HFpEF) 38, 39, 47, 77, 78, 92, 97, 98, 99, 119, 120, 127, 131, 160, 168 (fn), 178, 231, 232, 233, 234, 238, 267, 276, 278, 277, 280, 281

reduced, EF (HFrEF) 38, 39, 47, 67, 77, 78, 90, 127, 137, 138, 141, 143, 145, 147, 152, 156, 160, 161, 162, 168 (fn), 169, 174, 177, 193, 224, 231, 235, 267, 274, 276, 278, 279, 282

electrocardiogram (ECG) 56, 74, 75, 90, 106, 108, 162, 173, 174, 177, 206, 209, 210, 212, 244, 256, 262, 263, 272, 273, 278

empagliflozin 166, 167, 168 (fn), 197, 204 (fn), 278, 279

enalapril 141, 254, 274, 278, 281, 282

eplerenone 136, 137, 138, 140, 254, 274, 278

erythropoietin (EPO) 201, 278

extra corporeal membrane oxygenation (ECMO) 208, 278

F

fluid balance 35, 49, 54, 57, 58, 61, 62, 67, 81, 120, 128, 138, 139, 140, 141, 151, 153, 176, 197, 236, 243, 245, 248, 272, 278, 279, 280

fluid tablets
see diuretics

furosemide 75, 92, 99, 125, 130, 138, 140, 152, 207, 236, 254, 256, 278

G

gliflozin 130, 166, 167, 277, 278, 279, 282

glomerulus 51, 52, 57, 63, 66, 133, 134, 135, 141, 142, 147, 149, 151, 152, 160, 167, 258, 274, 278, 279, 280, 281

H

heart attack 8, 18(fn), 21, 85, 103,11, 127, 170, 184, 209, 210, 211, 212, 225, 274, 277, 279, 283, 286, 287

heart transplant/transplantation 78, 80, 131, 182, 184-188, 190, 209, 250, 251, 279

HFpEF, HFrEF
see ejection fraction

homeostasis 61, 62, 65, 69, 279

hibernating myocardium 86, 279

hydralazine 130, 159, 161, 168, 254, 279

I

implantable cardiac defibrillator (ICD) 131, 169, 170, 171, 173, 189, 239, 273, 279

incompetence
see leak

intra-aortic balloon pump (IABP) 208, 279

ivabradine 130, 159, 161, 165, 168, 254, 257, 279

K

Kerley B lines 107, 273, 279

kidneys 16, 17, 31, 32, 33, 35, 45, 48, 49, 51, 53, 54, 56, 57–70, 80, 83, 95, 107, 120, 129, 130, 133, 134-135, 136, 139, 145, 147, 149, 151, 152, 153, 154, 159, 166, 201, 208, 221, 236, 272, 275, 277, 278, 279, 280, 281, 282, 283

L

layers of the heart 44, 272, 280

leak/regurgitation/incompetence (valves) 93, 94, 115, 180, 181, 189, 273, 283

left atrium decompression 131, 178, 189, 280

left bundle branch block (LBBB) 90, 91, 162, 163, 174, 280

left ventricular assist device (LVAD) 183, 209, 250, 280

left ventricular function/dysfunction 77, 147, 156, 164, 166, 170, 193, 194, 209

Loop of Henle 63, 133, 135, 138-139, 140, 158, 278, 280

lungs 13, 17, 23, 28, 30, 32, 35, 41, 43, 46, 47, 48, 49, 53, 54, 56, 60, 64, 65, 66, 69, 77, 81, 82, 86, 88, 91, 95, 101, 105, 107,28, 129, 144, 157, 174, 176, 178, 189, 196, 205, 206, 207, 213, 223, 235, 241, 260, 272, 275, 276, 277, 279, 280, 281, 283, 284

J

juxtaglomerular apparatus 57, 133, 258, 280

M

metoprolol 156, 254, 257, 275, 277, 280, 281

mineralocorticoid 136, 139, 152, 274, 280

mineralocorticoid blocker 139, 152, 280

moxonidine 192, 280

myocardium 43, 44, 86, 88, 89, 116, 166, 168, 279, 280, 284

N

natriuretic peptide system (NPS)

nebivolol 156, 254, 275, 277, 280, 281

neprilysin inhibitor 130, 159-160, 165, 167, 218, 234, 250, 254, 281, 282

New York Heart Association Classification of Cardiac Failure (NYHA) *see cardiac failure, function*

nephron 52, 64, 134, 272, 281

neurohumoral 31, 32, 34, 243, 250, 281

nitrates 130, 159, 161, 168, 254, 281

non-steroid anti-inflammatory drug (NSAID) 151–153, 154, 198, 281

O

orthopnea 81, 82, 101, 282

P

paroxysmal nocturnal dyspnea (PND) 82, 101, 282

perindopril 141, 254, 274, 278, 281, 282

peripheral edema 102, 108, 281

porcine 252

potassium 107, 136, 138, 142, 143, 144, 145, 148, 153, 154, 255, 260, 281

preserved EF (HFpEF) *see ejection fraction*

pulmonary artery blood pressure monitoring 131, 176, 281

R

ramipril 92, 141, 164, 236, 254, 274, 278, 281, 282

receptors 58

regurgitation *see leak*

renin-angiotensin-aldosterone system (RAAS) 57, 62, 64, 65, 66, 68, 70, 130, 147, 150, 165, 250, 258, 272, 274, 280, 282

RAAS blocker 130, 250, 274, 282

reduced EF (HFrEF) *see ejection fraction*

respiratory system 41, 53, 54, 272, 277, 282

resynchronization therapy 131, 165, 173, 177, 189, 250, 279, 282

S

sacubitril 160, 234, 254, 257, 281, 282

salt/sodium 35, 49, 51, 54, 57, 58, 61, 62, 63, 64, 66, 67, 69, 79, 80, 83, 130, 131, 136, 138, 141, 142, 143, 144, 147, 154, 159, 166, 167, 168, 197, 222, 227, 250, 254, 255, 260, 274, 277, 278, 279, 280, 281, 282

shortness of breath 14, 15, 17, 26, 32, 33, 77, 79, 80, 81, 82, 86, 90, 91, 96, 97, 99, 101, 106, 108, 113, 119, 120, 121, 122, 129, 139, 143, 158, 164, 174, 179, 196, 198, 205, 206, 218, 221, 232, 233, 235, 236, 238, 245, 276, 278, 282

sodium-glucose transport inhibitor (SGLT2) 130, 159, 166-167, 168, 197, 277, 278, 279, 282

spironolactone 75, 92, 136, 137, 138, 140, 164, 242, 254, 256, 274, 282

stenosis 149, 180, 181, 273, 274, 275, 282, 283

stent/ing 97, 131, 170, 179, 184, 188 (fn), 189, 273, 276, 279, 280, 283

stroke 8, 21, 181, 192, 194, 203, 276, 277, 283

stroke volume 40

systole/systolic 36, 37, 38, 39, 40, 47, 77, 105,10,11, 269, 273, 277, 283, 278

T

takotsubo
see cardiomyopathy

transcutaneous aortic valve implantation (TAVI) 180, 181, 190, 283

troponin 162, 206, 210, 269, 283

U

ultrafiltration 208, 283

V

valsartan 147, 234, 254, 274, 276, 283

valve/s 8, 22, 28, 36, 41, 44, 46, 50, 51, 66, 68, 85, 93, 94, 103, 104,10, 113, 114, 115, 127, 128, 131, 134, 180-181, 189, 206, 209, 272, 273, 276, 278, 283

   aortic 23, 24, 28, 42, 44, 47, 61, 94, 163, 165, 180-181, 190, 273, 283

   aortic, bicuspid 162, 163, 165, 275

   aortic, tricuspid 163

   biological tissue/pig 180, 181, 189, 222, 223, 252, 283

   metallic 180, 181, 189, 283

   mitral 23, 24, 27, 28, 41, 44, 47, 94, 180, 189, 273, 283

   pulmonary 23, 24, 28, 94, 283

   tricuspid 23, 24, 27, 28, 43, 48, 94, 283

valve repair/replacement 131, 180, 190, 252, 283

vasoconstriction 31, 66, 67, 141, 143, 147, 159, 274, 283

vein/s 23, 28, 30, 42, 43, 45, 46, 47, 48, 52, 79, 103, 104, 179, 202, 203, 207, 276, 284
   deep vein thrombosis (DVT) 241, 276

   inferior vena cava (IVC) 16, 23, 24, 28, 30, 43, 45, 46, 48, 103, 178, 284

   jugular 55, 103, 104, 138, 284

   neck 98

   pulmonary 23, 24, 28, 41, 43, 47, 284

   renal 52, 135, 282

   superior vena cava (SVC) 23, 24, 28, 30, 43, 45, 46, 48, 103, 104, 138, 178, 284

ventricle/s 22, 23, 26, 27, 28, 91, 94, 105, 109, 162, 164, 170, 173, 175, 261, 277, 284

    right 23, 24, 28, 30, 43, 48, 87, 172, 176, 260, 275, 283, 284

    left/LV 23, 24, 25, 27, 28, 30, 35, 37, 39, 40, 41, 45, 47, 77, 85, 86, 87, 88, 93, 94, 98, 105, 109, 114, 128, 137, 138, 141, 143, 156, 159, 160, 162, 163, 164, 165, 170, 172, 174, 175, 177, 178, 191, 193, 206, 210, 211, 231, 260, 262, 275, 276, 278, 280, 281, 282, 283, 284

verapamil 192, 277, 284

viable heart muscle 85, 171, 284

X

xenograft / xenotransplantation 182, 190, 251, 284

Thanks

Cardiac Failure Explained would still be a good idea waiting to happen without the assistance, inspiration and backing from numerous people.

Among them are colleagues whom I hold in the highest regard and who were generous in finding precious time in their busy schedules to offer professional review and collegial encouragement. Special mention must be made of internationally respected **Professor Andrew Sidone** who is one of the lead authors for the Australian CCF guidelines. Not only did he suggest material that was valuable within the book, but he also generously provided the foreword. Another is **Doctor Michelle Kostner** who, as a discerning first-reader, asked probing questions, spotted weaknesses, and offered thoughtful suggestions. I would also like to acknowledge the contributors to the guideline papers that support this book. The guideline documents are enormous undertakings driven by colleagues donating their time for better medical care.

I am grateful to **my CF patients** who have contributed to my collective experience upon which I was able to base this book and especially to those whose case studies and personal journeys are used throughout its pages, bringing the often-complex CF medicinal theory into the realm of lived reality.

Invaluable and frank man-in-the-street-comments were received from the eagle-eyed masters of detail **David Thomas** and **John Harbinson.**

And then there are technical professionals who also helped create this book. Designer and artist **Cathy McAuliffe** has an overflowing abundance of creative capacity; **Beverly Waldie** is a master of the computer; **John North** and his unit expertly make the book available to you, the reader, and **Penny Edman,** a writer who works with me, is the best, bringing word-craft, single-mindedness, and passion to this highly talented team.

To these collaborators, to Chelle and my supportive family, and to everyone else involved in the production of *Cardiac Failure Explained,* I am truly grateful.

Warrick Bishop

About the authors

Warrick Bishop is a practising cardiologist with a passion for helping people live as well as possible for as long as possible. He has a special interest in preventing heart attack by using cardiac CT imaging, managing cholesterol and giving attention to diet. He also supports patients through education as he believes that the best-educated patients receive the best health care.

Warrick graduated from the University of Tasmania, School of Medicine, in 1988. He worked in the Northern Territory before undertaking his specialist training in Adelaide, South Australia. He completed his advanced training in cardiology in Hobart, Tasmania, becoming a fellow of the Royal Australian College of Physicians in 1997. He has worked predominantly in private practice.

In 2009, Warrick undertook training in CT cardiac coronary angiography, becoming the first cardiologist in Tasmania with this specialist recognition. This area of imaging fits well with his interest in preventative cardiology and was the focus of his first book, *Have You Planned Your Heart Attack?* (2016). He is a member of the Society of Cardiovascular Computed Tomography, Australian and New Zealand International Regional Committee (SCCT ANZ IRC).

Warrick is also a member of the Australian Atherosclerosis Society and a participant on the panel of 'interested parties' developing a model of care and a national registry for familial hypercholesterolemia. He has also developed a particular interest in diabetic-related-risk of coronary artery disease, specifically related to eating guidelines and lipid profiles.

Warrick is an accredited examiner for the Royal Australian College of Physicians and is regularly involved with teaching medical students and junior doctors. He has worked on projects, in an affiliate capacity, with Hobart's globally recognised Menzies Institute for Medical Research and has been recognised by the Medical School of the University of Tasmania with academic status.

A member of the Clinical Issues Committee of the Australian Heart Foundation which provides input into issues of significance for the management of heart patients, Warrick contributed to the Australian Heart Foundation's 2021 position paper on Coronary Artery Calcium.

Warrick enjoys a strong social media profile and in February 2020 he presented a TEDx talk, *Lessons from a Heart Attack*, at Docklands, Victoria, Australia, and then another soon after, *How Medicine, Money and Mindset are Costing Lives*, before a live audience at the University of Mississippi, Jackson, Mississippi, USA.

In addition to authoring numerous articles and the books, *Have You Planned Your Heart Attack?* (published in the USA as *Know Your Real Risk of Heart Attack*), *Atrial Fibrillation Explained* and now *Cardiac Failure Explained*, he founded the Healthy Heart Network in 2018.

All of Warrick's public endeavours are aimed at helping people live as well as possible for as long as possible by education and support.

A keen surfer, he enjoys travel and music and playing the guitar with his children.

Penelope Edman is a freelance writer, editor, high performance coach and photographer based in Hobart, Tasmania, Australia. After beginning her print journalism career in Bundaberg, Queensland, in the late 1970s, she moved to Hobart in 1991. She is an Australasian award-winning journalist and editor, and her articles and photographs have been published throughout Australia and internationally. She authored four non-fiction books before assisting Dr Bishop with *Have You Planned Your Heart Attack?*, *Atrial Fibrillation Explained* and *Cardiac Failure Explained*.

OTHER BOOKS FROM DOCTOR WARRICK BISHOP

#1 INTERNATIONAL BEST SELLER

ATRIAL FIBRILLATION *explained*

UNDERSTANDING THE NEXT CARDIAC EPIDEMIC

FOREWORD BY
PROFESSOR GARY JENNINGS

DOCTOR WARRICK BISHOP

#1 INTERNATIONAL BEST SELLER

Foreword by Professor Matthew J. Budoff M.D.

KNOW YOUR REAL RISK OF HEART ATTACK

Is The Single Biggest Killer Lurking In You
And What To Do About It

Dr Warrick Bishop

AS SEEN ON
60 MINUTES

Preface by Charles Wooley

ATRIAL FIBRILLATION Explained

It is very likely that you or someone you love is one of the 30 million people worldwide who has the 'irregularly irregular' heartbeat of atrial fibrillation.

An ageing population and our Western lifestyle are ensuring that the prevalence of atrial fibrillation, often referred to by its initials, AF, is increasing at such a rate that it is predicted to be the next cardiac epidemic. Despite it being so widespread, AF does not allow a one-treatment-for-all approach. While it can be managed, currently AF cannot be cured, so you could have it for a long time.

Atrial Fibrillation Explained is a must-read for sufferers and those who care about them, medical practitioners and anyone planning to live into a healthy, old age. Having a better understanding of AF as a disease and learning about its treatment will open up meaningful conversations between patients and their medical practitioners.

Available everywhere in Paperback, Hardcover, eBook and AudioBook including
https://drwarrickbishop.com/page/books

Know Your Real Risk of HEART ATTACK

A number of years ago something incredible, an amazing coincidence, happened that started Warrick on the mission to prevent heart attacks rather than try to cure them. He was driving to work one day when he stopped at a commotion by the side of the road. A fun runner had collapsed during a fun run with a heart attack. He helped in his resuscitation only to find out that had seen the very same man two years earlier and reassured him that he was fine.

Warrick had missed the chance to make a difference and it nearly cost a life!! . Based on risk calculation and the best practice of the time, he shouldn't have been at high risk.....but he was!

This important question started him on a journey which meant he was open to looking more closely at new and emerging technology to help in being more precise about risk of heart attack.

Available everywhere in Paperback, Hardcover, eBook and AudioBook including
https://drwarrickbishop.com/page/books

CPSIA information can be obtained
at www.ICGtesting.com
Printed in the USA
LVHW080018180822
726258LV00014B/874